THE VACCINE HANDBOOK

THE VACCINE HANDBOOK

A Practitioner's Guide to Maximizing Use and Efficacy across the Lifespan

SECOND EDITION

Tina Q. Tan, MD, John P. Flaherty, MD, and Daniel P. Dunham, MD, MPH

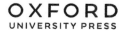

OXFORD
UNIVERSITY PRESS

Oxford University Press is a department of the University of Oxford.
It furthers the University's objective of excellence in research, scholarship,
and education by publishing worldwide. Oxford is a registered trade mark of
Oxford University Press in the UK and certain other countries.

Published in the United States of America by Oxford University Press
198 Madison Avenue, New York, NY 10016, United States of America.

© Oxford University Press 2025

All rights reserved. No part of this publication may be reproduced, stored in a retrieval system, transmitted, used for text and data mining, or used for training artificial intelligence, in any form or by any means, without the prior permission in writing of Oxford University Press, or as expressly permitted by law, by license or under terms agreed with the appropriate reprographics rights organization. Inquiries concerning reproduction outside the scope of the above should be sent to the Rights Department, Oxford University Press, at the address above.

You must not circulate this work in any other form
and you must impose this same condition on any acquirer

Library of Congress Cataloging-in-Publication Data
Names: Tan, Tina Q. author | Flaherty, John P. author | Dunham, Daniel P. author
Title: The vaccine handbook / Tina Q. Tan, John P. Flaherty, Daniel P. Dunham.
Description: Second edition. | New York, NY, United States of America :
Oxford University Press, 2025. | Includes bibliographical references and index. |
Identifiers: LCCN 2024032081 | ISBN 9780197792933 cp |
ISBN 9780197792957 epub
Subjects: LCSH: Vaccines—Handbooks, manuals, etc. |
LCGFT: Handbooks and manuals
Classification: LCC RA638 .T35 2025 | DDC 614.4/7—dc23/eng/20241112
LC record available at https://lccn.loc.gov/2024032081

This material is not intended to be, and should not be considered, a substitute for medical or other professional advice. Treatment for the conditions described in this material is highly dependent on the individual circumstances. And, while this material is designed to offer accurate information with respect to the subject matter covered and to be current as of the time it was written, research and knowledge about medical and health issues is constantly evolving and dose schedules for medications are being revised continually, with new side effects recognized and accounted for regularly. Readers must therefore always check the product information and clinical procedures with the most up-to-date published product information and data sheets provided by the manufacturers and the most recent codes of conduct and safety regulation. The publisher and the authors make no representations or warranties to readers, express or implied, as to the accuracy or completeness of this material. Without limiting the foregoing, the publisher and the authors make no representations or warranties as to the accuracy or efficacy of the drug dosages mentioned in the material. The authors and the publisher do not accept, and expressly disclaim, any responsibility for any liability, loss, or risk that may be claimed or incurred as a consequence of the use and/or application of any of the contents of this material.

DOI: 10.1093/med/9780197792933.001.0001

Printed by Integrated Books International, United States of America

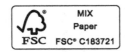

CONTENTS

Introduction ix

PART I. VACCINE OVERVIEW 1

Vaccine Facts 1

Addressing Patient Concerns About Receiving Vaccines 3

Common Vaccines by Type 19

Administering Vaccines: Dose, Route, Site, and Needle Size 19

PART II. VACCINES THROUGHOUT THE LIFE CYCLE 25

2024 Infant, Child, and Adolescent Immunization Schedules 26

CONTENTS

2024 Adult Immunization Schedules	37
Summary of Vaccines Routinely Recommended for Infants, Children, and Adults	46
Vaccines and Pregnancy	58

PART III. ROUTINE VACCINES FOR VACCINE-PREVENTABLE DISEASES 73

Diphtheria	73
Tetanus	78
Pertussis	85
Influenza	98
Hepatitis A	117
Hepatitis B	125
Measles	134
Mumps	141
Rubella	145
Varicella Zoster (Chickenpox)	152
Herpes Zoster (Shingles)	164
Pneumococcal Disease	171
Meningococcal Disease	182
Human Papillomavirus	194

Hemophilus influenzae Type b Disease	201
Poliovirus Infections	208
Rotavirus Infections	216
Contraindications and Precautions to Commonly Used Vaccines	223
COVID-19	228
Respiratory Syncytial Virus	235
Dengue	243
Mpox	247

PART IV. TRAVEL VACCINES — 255

Yellow Fever Vaccine	255
Typhoid Fever Vaccine	260
Japanese Encephalitis Vaccine	265
Rabies Vaccine	270
Cholera Vaccine	276
Tick-Borne Encephalitis Vaccine	282

Index	289

INTRODUCTION

DID YOU KNOW THAT:

- The concept of vaccination and attempts to vaccinate has been traced back to the 7th century when some Indian Buddhists drank snake venom in an attempt to become immune to its effects.
- Immunization is one of the most successful public health initiatives of all time. Each year, immunization prevents an estimated 2 to 3 million deaths from diphtheria, tetanus, pertussis, and measles worldwide. These are all life-threatening diseases that disproportionately affect children.
- Immunization was critical in the eradication of smallpox and the near eradication of polio.
- One out of five infants worldwide (20% of children) remains unprotected against common vaccine-preventable diseases—more than 70% live in 10 countries: Afghanistan,

INTRODUCTION

Chad, the Democratic Republic of Congo, Ethiopia, India, Indonesia, Nigeria, Pakistan, the Philippines, and South Africa.

The development of vaccines against multiple infectious diseases is one of the greatest public health achievements of the past century. Infant and childhood vaccination rates are high in the United States; however, vaccination rates in the adolescent and the adult populations are still below the Healthy People 2030 goals, leaving much room for improvement. Vaccine-preventable diseases (VPDs) still cause 50,000 to 90,000 deaths and hundreds of thousands of hospitalizations in adults each year in the United States. This poses a major public health problem to everyone in the community, especially to young infants who are either too young to be immunized or incompletely immunized. To protect against these VPDs, an increasing number of preventative vaccines are recommended for routine administration to persons of all ages.

So what makes this book different? This book covers the majority of vaccine issues and provides answers to common questions that a busy health care provider may encounter on a daily basis presented in a practical, easy-to-read, and easy-to-understand format. The book can easily be carried in a lab coat pocket or can be quickly accessed from office or clinic shelves to provide ready answers to common issues. The book is written so that health care providers in different specialties and at all levels of training and practice can optimally recommend the appropriate vaccines for their patients of any age. There are several comprehensive textbooks covering all aspects of vaccinology in great detail, but these books are not formatted as a quick, readily accessible reference while seeing patients in an office, clinic, or on patient rounds.

INTRODUCTION

Today, the practice of medicine requires health care providers to obtain and record more comprehensive patient information, including complete vaccination histories on their patients. This book not only is written to assist all providers in obtaining vaccine histories but also provides guidance in recommending and administering the currently recommended vaccines for age according to Centers for Disease Control and Prevention guidelines. In addition, the book has a section on addressing and speaking with vaccine-hesitant patients, which is an issue that is being encountered more frequently by health care providers in all areas of medicine. Storage and procedural issues are well covered in the book, and the book provides guidance for health care providers taking care of patients of any age.

As our world shrinks and international travel becomes easier, more widespread, and affordable, many VPDs which are still endemic in other countries are now just a plane, boat, car, or bus ride away. Individuals who travel to these countries and are not appropriately vaccinated can contract these diseases and become ill while traveling or bring the disease back home, serving as a nidus for spread to other citizens. This handbook provides guidance to the health care provider in preparing patients who are planning to travel to countries abroad to protect them against various diseases.

Also, the "Did You Know That" sections at the beginning of each chapter provide interesting and light-hearted information about the vaccines and VPDs.

A major barrier to vaccine usage, especially in the adult population, is a widespread lack of understanding among health care providers caring primarily for adults concerning

- the importance of preventative vaccines in their patients;
- the diseases against which the preventative vaccines provide protection;

INTRODUCTION

- the population for whom the vaccines are indicated;
- cost issues and reimbursement; and
- responsibility for providing vaccine information and vaccine access to their patients.

Solutions to these barriers are addressed in the book.

We invite you to explore this practical and easy-to-understand handbook and hope that you will find the information useful in gaining a better understanding of why preventative vaccination should be an integral part of routine health care at all ages, providing some suggestions to help you talk to your patients about vaccines, and arming you with the information needed so that you can provide the recommended vaccinations to them.

We look forward to any thoughts and suggestions that you may have in helping us improve this handbook.

Tina Q. Tan, MD
John P. Flaherty, MD
Daniel P. Dunham, MD, MPH

PART I

VACCINE OVERVIEW

VACCINE FACTS

- **Active immunization** involves the administration of all or part of a microorganism or a modified product of a microorganism (a toxoid, a purified antigen, or an antigen produced by genetic engineering) to evoke an immunologic response that mimics that of natural infection.
- **Passive immunization** involves the administration of preformed antibody to a recipient and achieves protection only for a short period of time (intramuscular [IM] immunoglobulin or intravenous immunoglobulin [IVIG]).
- Vaccines may be **inactivated** or **live, attenuated**. Inactivated vaccines are composed of inactivated whole cells or particles that are unable to multiply. These vaccines function by stimulating humoral immune responses and by priming for immunological memory. With live, attenuated vaccines, there is active replication of the organism in the host that produces a modified infection to which the host develops an immune response.

- Vaccine dose administration is based on the **age** of the person, unlike other medications that are dosed by weight or body surface area.
- The **immunologic response to a vaccine** is dependent on the type and dose of antigen; the effect of adjuvants (materials added to a vaccine to improve the immune response to the antigen [e.g., aluminum salts]); and host factors related to age, preexisting antibody, nutrition, concurrent disease, immune status, or drug effect and genetics of the host.
- Vaccines are developed with the smallest dose of antigen that will elicit a robust immune response with the lowest side effect profile.
- Some vaccines provide nearly complete and lifelong protection against disease, others provide partial protection, and some need to be given at regular intervals to maintain disease protection.
- Two or more inactivated vaccines may be administered simultaneously in different sites.
- Inactivated and live vaccines may be administered simultaneously (tetanus, diphtheria, acellular pertussis [Tdap] and intranasal influenza).
- Two or more live vaccines may be administered simultaneously at the **same** visit.
- A **break** in the **immunization schedule of a vaccine** does **not** require **starting the entire series over** or **giving additional doses** of the vaccine. If a dose of vaccine is missed, subsequent immunization should be given at the next visit as if the usual interval between doses had elapsed.

- **Live, attenuated vaccines** are **contraindicated** in persons who are **pregnant** and those **with known or suspected immunodeficiency** (there are some exceptions).

The Advisory Committee on Immunization Practices (ACIP) of the Centers for Disease Control and Prevention (CDC) now designates a **vaccine recommendation as either "A" or "B"**:

- An "A" recommendation means the vaccine is routinely recommended for all children and adults in an age or risk group.
- A "B" recommendation means that the vaccine is for permissive use at the discretion of the clinician or health care provider with shared clinical decision-making between the health care provider and patient.

The Affordable Care Act requires insurance plans to provide benefit coverage of vaccines with both A and B recommendations. The Vaccines for Children program also includes vaccines with a B recommendation.

ADDRESSING PATIENT CONCERNS ABOUT RECEIVING VACCINES

Vaccines are one of the greatest public health achievements of modern medicine. In the early 20th century, before the routine use of vaccines, about one in six children younger than age 5 years died of a vaccine-preventable disease, especially diseases such as measles, smallpox, pertussis, or rubella. Vaccination programs have contributed significantly to the marked decline in morbidity and mortality of various vaccine-preventable diseases and are credited with the worldwide eradication of smallpox and the virtual elimination of polio from many areas of the world. However, concerns about the safety of vaccines and hesitancy to receive vaccines have been voiced since the introduction of vaccines to the public. For example, Benjamin Franklin's son, Francis Folger Franklin, died at age 4 years of smallpox. The following is a quote from Franklin expressing his profound regret for not immunizing his son and his advice to parents regarding vaccination:

> In 1736 I lost one of my sons, a fine boy of four years old, by the smallpox, taken in the common way. I long regretted bitterly, and still regret that I had not given it to him by inoculation. This I mention for the sake of parents who omit that operation, on the supposition that they should never forgive themselves if a child died under it; my example showing that the regret may be the same either way, and that, therefore, the safer should be chosen.

There is a plethora of information on vaccine safety that is available from multiple sources. As patients search the internet for information on vaccines, they frequently encounter information from poorly designed and conducted studies, misleading information from well-conducted studies, anecdotes, or personal testimonies that are incorrectly written or written to look like real science and that claim vaccines cause autism and are associated with experimentation, are not effective, and in many cases are associated with devastating side effects. Addressing these concerns and fears during a routine health evaluation may be time-consuming and stressful for both the health care provider and the patient (Table 1). Health care providers play a key role in establishing and maintaining a commitment to effectively communicating with

Table 1 BARRIERS TO ADOLESCENT AND ADULT IMMUNIZATION

Patient Barriers	Physician Barriers
• Lack of awareness of disease and associated morbidity	• Lack of organized vaccine administration infrastructure
• Perception that vaccine has no value and is ineffective	• Lack of understanding of importance of vaccines
• Perception of low risk for disease	• Lack of understanding of the diseases the vaccines protect against and the population for whom vaccines are recommended
• Perception that vaccines are experimental and may be dangerous	
• Lack of access to vaccines	• Lack of awareness of vaccine recommendations
• Immunization costs	• Discomfort using vaccines
• Requirement for multiple doses	• Missed opportunities and patient refusal
• Perceived vaccine risks and fears of side effects (e.g., developing autism)	• Time limitations and patient refusal
• Lack of vaccination records	• Perception that it is another primary health care provider's responsibility
• Time limitations	• Vaccine costs and reimbursement
• Perception that getting natural disease is better than receiving vaccine	• Inability to verify previous vaccination records
	• Storage requirements

patients about the importance of vaccines and maintaining high vaccination rates. We must remember that a successful discussion about vaccines involves a two-way conversation, with both parties sharing information and asking questions. Important principles to bring to the discussion include taking time to listen (this can play a major role in helping patients with their decisions to choose vaccination) and soliciting and welcoming questions and concerns—these simple principles go a long way in connecting with patients and facilitating a productive dialogue.

Studies have shown that most adults do believe that vaccines are important, and a health care provider's recommendation is the critical factor in whether patients receive the vaccines that they and/or their children need. Recommendation of a vaccine by a health care provider prompts most patients to get immunized.

However, for some patients, a strong, clear vaccine recommendation may not be enough. The health care provider can encourage these patients to make an informed decision about vaccination by sharing critical information with them. Based on the CDC SHARE program, the following steps should be included in discussing vaccines with these patients:

1. **Sharing** the reasons why the recommended vaccine is appropriate for the patient based on their age, health status, lifestyle, occupation, or other factors that place them at risk for a disease
2. **Highlighting** positive experiences with vaccines to reinforce the benefits and strengthen confidence in vaccination
3. **Addressing** all patient questions and concerns about the vaccine, including potential side effects, safety, and vaccine effectiveness, in easy-to-understand language

4. **Reminding** patients that vaccines protect them and their families from many common and serious diseases
5. **Explaining** the potential costs associated with getting the disease, including serious complications, time lost from missing work or family obligations, and the financial costs

The following are common misconceptions regarding vaccines that patients may express and strategies for addressing these issues.

Misconception #1: Vaccines cause autism

The widespread fear that vaccines increased the risk for autism originated with a 1997 study published in *The Lancet* by Andrew Wakefield, a British gastroenterologist. His study in a small number of children suggested that measles, mumps, rubella (MMR) vaccine was the cause of the increasing amount of autism that was being seen in British children. Further scientific review of the data led to the paper being completely discredited, and the paper was retracted due to serious procedural errors, ethical violations, false reporting of data, and undisclosed financial conflicts of interest. Ultimately, Wakefield lost his medical license. However, his hypothesis (which is completely false) continues to be taken seriously by people in the community. Multiple major studies have been conducted, and none have found a link between any vaccine and the likelihood of developing autism.

The issue of whether vaccines cause autism spectrum disorder (ASD) has been studied extensively, including several very thorough reviews by the Institute of Medicine (IOM). A 2004 scientific review by IOM concluded that "the evidence favors rejection of a causal relationship between thimerosal-containing vaccines and ASD." Since 2003, there have been nine CDC-funded or -conducted studies that have found no link between thimerosal-containing vaccines and ASD and no link between the MMR vaccine and ASD in children. In 2011, an IOM report on eight routinely used vaccines (MMR, hepatitis A, meningococcal, varicella zoster, influenza, hepatitis B, human papillomavirus, and tetanus containing vaccines) given to children and adults found that these vaccines are very safe and that there is no link between receiving vaccines and developing ASD. A 2013 CDC study added to the research showing that vaccines do not cause ASD. The study examined the number of antigens (substances in vaccines that cause the body's immune system to produce disease-fighting antibodies) from vaccines during the first 2 years of life. The results showed that the total amount of antigen from vaccines received was the same between children with ASD and those who did not have ASD. All the extensive research performed to date shows absolutely no evidence of any link between receiving vaccines or those vaccines containing trace thimerosal and ASD.

The true causes of autism are probably multifactorial but have no link to vaccines. Several recent studies have identified symptoms of autism in children well before they receive the MMR vaccine, and others provide evidence that autism may develop in utero well before the infant is born or receives any vaccines.

Health Care Provider Communication Tips

When patients raise concerns and hypotheses linking vaccines to autism, there are four items critical in addressing these issues:

1. The health care provider should provide the patient with empathetic reassurance that they understand that the patient's health or their child's health is the patient's top priority and that it is also the health care provider's top priority to ensure that putting the patient or their child at

risk of vaccine-preventable diseases without any scientific evidence of a link between vaccines and autism is a risk that the health care provider is not willing to take.
2. Acknowledge that the onset of symptoms of ASD is known to often coincide with the timing of vaccines but is in no way caused by vaccines. Offer to share information from well-designed and well-conducted studies that show that MMR and other vaccines do not cause autism.
3. Emphasize that as a health care provider, your personal and professional opinion is that vaccines are very safe and are important in protecting against potentially serious infections.
4. Remind the patient that vaccine-preventable diseases may cause serious complications and even death and that these diseases are still present and remain a threat.

Misconception #2: An infant's immune system becomes overwhelmed and cannot handle the number of vaccines given

Infant immune systems are much stronger than one might imagine. Neonates develop the capacity to respond to foreign antigens before they are born. B and T cells are present by 14 weeks' gestation and express an enormous array of antigen-specific receptors. Based on the number of antibodies present in the blood, an infant would theoretically have the ability to respond to approximately 10,000 vaccines at one time. So even if all the doses of the scheduled vaccines during the first 5 years of life were given at once, it would only "use up" approximately 0.1% (1/10th of 1%) of an infant's immune capacity. The immune system can never really be overwhelmed given that the cells in the system are constantly being replenished (e.g., 2 billion CD4$^+$ T lymphocytes are replenished on a daily basis). In reality, infants are exposed to tens of thousands of bacteria and viruses on a daily basis through the activities of daily living in their environment (e.g., day care, going to the park, the grocery store, the mall, playdates, etc.), and the number of antigens in routine immunizations is negligible in comparison.

Health Care Provider Communication Tips
Parents/patients may bring up concerns of receiving more than one vaccine at a time, having a strong preference of receiving vaccines at a later time, and/or receiving vaccines on an alternative schedule with regard to timing and spacing of vaccines that is different from the recommended schedule. It is important to emphasize the following:

a. The routine vaccine schedules are designed to provide protection at the earliest possible time against serious diseases that may affect a person early in life. The timing of when the vaccines are administered in the routine schedule has been extensively studied and provides the optimal immune protection against a disease. Using alternative schedules is very strongly discouraged because it is unknown if a person will develop protective immunity against a disease by receiving vaccines by these schedules.

b. Vaccine-preventable diseases may be associated with serious morbidity and mortality that are prevented by vaccines.

c. Each vaccine series should be started on time to protect patients (especially infants and children) as soon as possible, and each multidose series must be completed to provide the best protection against a disease. Receiving only one dose of a multidose series does not provide adequate protective immunity.

Misconception #3: Natural immunity is better than vaccine-acquired immunity, and vaccines are more dangerous than the diseases they prevent

Most people have not learned firsthand of the threat of vaccine-preventable diseases because of the effectiveness of the vaccines that are used today. Therefore, many people assume that some diseases are no longer present and question whether vaccines are really needed. They may also believe that the risks of being vaccinated far outweigh the benefits of protecting them from infection caused by vaccine-preventable diseases.

In a small number of cases, natural immunity—defined as actually contracting the disease and becoming ill—may result in a stronger immune response to the disease than a vaccination. However, the dangers of this approach far outweigh any possible relative benefits. For example, if you wanted to develop immunity to measles by contracting the disease, you have a 1 in 500 chance of dying from your disease. In contrast, the number of people who have had severe allergic reactions from an MMR vaccine is less than 1 in 1 million. Likewise, a natural chickenpox infection may result in pneumonia, bacterial skin infections, or necrotizing fasciitis, whereas the varicella vaccine may only cause a sore arm or leg for a couple of days.

Health Care Provider Communication Tips
 a. Provide information from your own experience about the seriousness of the vaccine-preventable diseases (e.g., complications from influenza, pneumococcal disease, varicella, and herpes zoster).
 b. Explain that there continue to be cases and outbreaks of vaccine-preventable diseases occurring in the United

States, and that even when diseases have been eliminated in the United States, they still pose an important threat in unimmunized infants, children, and adults when traveling abroad or if they are exposed to an unimmunized person who travels abroad, contracts the disease, and brings it back to the United States.

c. Any vaccine-preventable disease can strike at any time in the United States because all of these diseases still circulate either in the United States or elsewhere in the world. A vaccine-preventable disease is only a plane, train, bus, boat, or car ride away.

Misconception #4: Vaccines contain harmful toxins

Fears over the safety of vaccines have substantially increased during the past three decades. Concerns have grown over the use of formaldehyde, mercury, or aluminum in vaccines. It is true that high levels of these chemicals are toxic to the human body; however, only minute trace amounts of some of these chemicals are used in U.S. Food and Drug Administration (FDA)–approved vaccines. For example, the amount of formaldehyde produced by our own metabolic systems is much higher than that used in vaccines, and there is no evidence that low levels of this chemical, mercury, or aluminum in vaccines are harmful.

Questions regarding the safety of thimerosal in vaccines continue to arise. Thimerosal contains a mercury compound that has been used widely as a preservative since the 1930s in a number of biological and drug products, including multidose vials of vaccines, to help prevent potentially life-threatening contamination with harmful microbes. Mercury is a naturally occurring element found in the environment. Certain bacteria can change mercury to methylmercury, which can make its way through the food chain in fish, animals, and humans. At high levels, methylmercury can be toxic to humans. Thimerosal contains a different organomercurial compound—ethylmercury. Ethylmercury is broken down and excreted much more rapidly than methylmercury and is unlikely to accumulate in the body and cause harm. Nevertheless, because of an increasing awareness of the theoretical potential for neurotoxicity of low levels of organomercurials, and the number of thimerosal-containing vaccines that had been added to the infant immunization schedule, the FDA elected to work with vaccine manufacturers to reduce or completely eliminate thimerosal from vaccines.

Thimerosal has been removed from or reduced to trace amounts (remaining as a part of the manufacturing process and defined as 1 µg or less of organomercury per dose) in all vaccines routinely recommended for children aged 6 years or younger, with the exception of a specific influenza vaccine. Preservative-free versions of the inactivated influenza vaccine and tetanus and diphtheria (Td) vaccine (both of which contain trace amounts of thimerosal) are available.

Table 2 shows vaccines in multidose vials that contain some thimerosal.

Health Care Provider Communication Tips
  a. Remind patients that there are ongoing efforts by the CDC and FDA to ensure the safety of the vaccines that are currently used and that the vaccines used today are the safest that they have ever been.
  b. Explain that in multiple studies, the various ingredients contained in vaccines (e.g., thimerosal, aluminum, gelatin,

Table 2 VACCINES CONTAINING THIMEROSAL (ONLY MULTIDOSE VIALS)

Vaccine	Brand	Manufacturer	Thimerosal Concentration (%)	Mercury (μg/0.5 mL)
Tetanus toxoid	Generic	Sanofi Pasteur	0.01	25
Influenza inactivated	Afluria	CSL limited for Merck	0.01	24.5
	FluLaval Quadrivalent	GlaxoSmithKline	0.01	25
	Fluvirin	Novartis	0.01	25
	Fluzone	Sanofi Pasteur	0.01	25

human serum albumin, formaldehyde, antibiotics, egg proteins, and yeast proteins) have not been found to be harmful in humans or experimental animals. The contents of these agents are minute and are used to prevent bacterial or fungal contamination (e.g., thimerosal), enhance antigen-specific immune responses (e.g., aluminum salts), stabilized live, attenuated viral vaccines (e.g., gelatin and human serum albumin), or are residuals from the manufacturing process (e.g., formaldehyde, antibiotics, egg proteins, and yeast proteins).

c. Use motivational interviewing techniques in which you resist telling patients what to do; seek to understand their values, needs, and motivation; listen with empathy; and empower them.

REFERENCES

1. Institute for Vaccine Safety. www.vaccinesafety.edu
2. Centers for Disease Control and Prevention. Thimerosal and vaccines. n.d. https://www.cdc.gov/vaccine-safety/about/thimerosal.html?CDC_AAref_Val=https://www.cdc.gov/vaccinesafety/concerns/thimerosal
3. U.S. Food and Drug Administration. Thimerosal in vaccines. n.d. https://www.fda.gov/vaccines-blood-biologics/safety-availability-biologics/thimerosal-and-vaccines
4. National Foundation for Infectious Diseases. Immunization. n.d. https://www.nfid.org/immunization
5. Hall K, Gibbie T, Lubman DI. Motivational interviewing techniques: Facilitating behaviour change in the general practice setting. *Aust Fam Physician*. 2012;41(9):660–667.
6. Best M, Katamba A, Neuhauser D. Making the right decision: Benjamin Franklin's son dies of smallpox in 1736. *Qual Saf Health Care*. 2007;16:478–480.
7. Institute of Medicine (US). Immunization Safety Review Committee. Immunization Safety Review: Vaccines and Autism, Washington, DC: National Academies Press US; 2004. PMID 20669467.
8. Institute of Medicine (US). Immunization Safety Review: Adverse Effects of Vaccines - Evidence and Causality. Washington, DC: National Academic Press US; 2011.
9. DeStefano F, Price CS, Weintraub ES. Increasing exposure to antibody-stimulating proteins and polysaccharides in vaccines is not associated with risk of autism. *J Pediatrics*. 2013, Mar 29.

Misconception #5: The development of better hygiene and sanitation, nutrition, and the development of antibiotics are responsible for decreasing the number of vaccine-preventable infections—not the vaccines themselves

Improved hygiene and sanitation, nutrition, and antibiotics have certainly all contributed to reducing rates of infectious diseases; however, when these factors are taken in isolation, their impact on the rates of vaccine-preventable infectious diseases is low compared to when vaccines are factored into the equation. The routine use of vaccines has had a substantial impact on the incidence of vaccine-preventable diseases and has resulted in the eradication of smallpox worldwide. A notable example of the impact of vaccination is the *Haemophilus influenzae* type b vaccine (Hib). Prior to the introduction of effective Hib conjugate vaccines in the early 1990s, Hib was the most common case of bacterial meningitis and invasive bacterial disease in the United States in children younger than age 5 years. In 1990, there were 20,000 cases of invasive Hib disease. Following the introduction of the vaccine, this number markedly declined to approximately 1,500 cases in 1993. With routine use of conjugate Hib vaccines, the incidence of Hib disease has decreased by 99% to fewer than 1 case per 100,000 children younger than age 5 years (or less than 50 cases per year). There were no significant changes in hygiene, sanitation, and nutrition during this time period. Currently in the United States, invasive Hib disease occurs primarily in unimmunized or underimmunized children and among infants too young to have completed the primary immunization series. Hib remains an important pathogen in many resource-limited countries in which Hib vaccines are not routinely available.

Health Care Provider Communication Tip
a. Provide some of the above information to your patients so that they have an understanding of the role that vaccines play in reducing and eliminating the incidence of vaccine preventable diseases.

Misconception #6: Vaccines are not worth the risk

Despite parental concerns, children have been successfully vaccinated for decades. There has never been a single credible study linking vaccines to long-term health conditions. It is also important for the patient to realize that by not being vaccinated, they place themself and/or their children at risk for contracting a vaccine-preventable disease that may have serious consequences. Patients need to be aware that the presentation of these diseases can range from mild to severe and life-threatening, and there is no way to know beforehand if a person will get a mild or serious case.

As long as a large majority (85% to 99%) of people are immunized in any population (herd immunity), even the unimmunized minority will be protected against a disease. This prevents a disease from being transmitted and spreading within the population. This is important because there will always be a portion of the population—young infants, pregnant women, elderly, and those with immunocompromising conditions—that cannot receive vaccines. However, if too many people fail to vaccinate themselves or their children, they contribute to an increasing danger that creates opportunities for viruses and bacteria to reestablish themselves in a community and spread. For example, international travel is rapidly growing. Even if a disease is not a threat in the United States, it may be common in other countries that do not routinely vaccinate against the disease. If someone from one of these countries were to carry the disease into the United States from abroad, or if an unvaccinated individual were to travel to that country and contract the disease, other unvaccinated individuals in the United States would be at a far greater risk of getting sick if they were exposed.

Health Care Provider Communication Tips
When patients make the decision to delay or reject vaccines, they need to understand that this can have a significant impact on their life, their child's life, or the life of someone else. They need to understand the following:

a. If they are ill or their child is ill and they visit the doctor, clinic, or a hospital emergency room, call 911, or ride in an ambulance, they must inform the medical staff that they or their child is unvaccinated or has not received all the recommended age-specific vaccines.
b. Telling health care personnel their vaccination status or their child's vaccination status is critical for several reasons:
   i. The treating physician will need to consider the possibility that the person has a vaccine-preventable disease as the cause of their illness.
   ii. The persons helping that patient or their child can take precautions (e.g., the patient can be placed in isolation) so that the disease does not spread to others, especially patients in high-risk groups that are either too young to be vaccinated or cannot be vaccinated due to an underlying condition.

Misconception #7: Vaccines can cause the disease and infection that they are trying to prevent

Vaccines can cause mild symptoms that may resemble those of the disease they are protecting against. A common misconception is that these symptoms indicate an infection when, in fact, in the small percentage of cases in which patients develop symptoms after the vaccine, it is the patient's own immune response to the vaccine and not an infection that is causing the symptoms.

Health Care Provider Communication Tips
If your patients are searching the internet for basic information on vaccines, recommend they seek websites that have a credible

source; whose information is updated on a regular basis; and whose content is researched, written, and approved by subject matter experts, including physicians, researchers, epidemiologists, and analysts. Reliable sources of vaccine information that you can use and direct your patient to include the following:

   a. American Academy of Pediatrics (https://www.aap.org/en/patient-care/immunizations/?srsltid=AfmBOoqwSuxrT9apvi5fAlB4DDocifHEI-G0n6Bq7QhH8HS19EZJinBg)
   b. Immunization Action Coalition (http://www.vaccineinformation.org/internet-immunization-info)
   c. National Network for Immunization Information (http://www.immunizationinfo.org/parents/evaluating-information-web)
   d. Medical Library Association (http://www.mlanet.org)

COMMON VACCINES BY TYPE

Table 3 shows the different vaccines by type.

ADMINISTERING VACCINES: DOSE, ROUTE, SITE, AND NEEDLE SIZE

Table 4 shows the different vaccine routes of administration, and Table 5 shows the different injection sites and needle size used for administration

Table 3 COMMON VACCINES BY TYPE

Inactivated Vaccines	Live, Attenuated Vaccines
Td (tetanus and diphtheria)	MMR (measles, mumps, rubella)
Tdap (tetanus, diphtheria, acellular pertussis)	Varicella
Injectable influenza	Intranasal influenza
Hepatitis A	Rotavirus (infants)
Hepatitis B	Oral typhoid fever
HPV (human papillomavirus)	Yellow fever
Haemophilus influenzae type b (Hib)	Oral cholera
IPV (inactivated poliovirus)	Dengue
Pneumococcal polysaccharide (PPSV23)	Mpox
Pneumococcal conjugate (PCV)	
Meningococcal conjugate (MCV4)	
Meningococcal B	
Injectable typhoid fever	
Japanese encephalitis	
Rabies	
Herpes zoster (Shingrix)	
COVID-19	
RSV	
Tick-borne encephalitis vaccine (TicoVax)	
Ebola	

VACCINE OVERVIEW

Table 4 ADMINISTERING VACCINES: DOSE AND ROUTE

Vaccine	Dose	Route of Administration
COVID-19	0.3 mL	IM
Diphtheria, tetanus, pertussis (DTaP, DT, Tdap, Td)	0.5 mL	IM
Dengue	0.5 mL	SC
Haemophilus influenzae type b (Hib)	0.5 mL	IM
Hepatitis A (Hep A)	≤18 years: 0.5 mL ≥19 years: 1.0 mL	IM
Hepatitis B (Hep B)	≤19 years: 0.5 mL ≥20 years: 1.0 mL	IM
Human papillomavirus (HPV)	0.5 mL	IM
Influenza: live, attenuated (LAIV)	0.2 mL (0.1 mL in each nostril)	Intranasal spray
Influenza: inactivated (IIV); recombinant (RIV) for ages 18 years or older	6 to 35 months: 0.25 mL ≥3 years: 0.5 mL	IM
Influenza: inactivated (IIV); intradermal for ages 18 through 64 years	0.1 mL	ID
Measles, mumps, rubella (MMR)	0.5 mL	SC

(continued)

Table 4 CONTINUED

Vaccine	Dose	Route of Administration
Meningococcal conjugate (MCV4 [MenACWY])	0.5 mL	IM
Meningococcal serogroup B (MenB)	0.5 mL	IM
Meningococcal conjugate pentavalent vaccine (MenABCWY)	0.5 mL	IM
Mpox (Jynneos)	0.5 mL	SC
	0.1 mL	ID
Pneumococcal conjugate (PCV)	0.5 mL	IM
Pneumococcal polysaccharide (PPSV23)	0.5 mL	IM or SC
Polio, inactivated (IPV)	0.5 mL	IM or SC
Respiratory syncytial virus (RSV) long acting monoclonal antibody	≤5 kg: 0.5 mL	IM
	>5 kg: 1.0 mL	IM
RSV PreF3 vaccine (adjuvanted)	0.5 mL	IM
RSV preF vaccine	0.5 mL	
Rotavirus (RV)	Rotarix (RV1): 1.0 mL	Oral
	Rotateq (RV5): 2.0 mL	
Tick-borne encephalitis vaccine (TicoVax)	0.5 mL	IM
Varicella	0.5 mL	SC

Table 4 CONTINUED

Vaccine	Dose	Route of Administration
Zoster	0.5 mL	IM
Combination vaccines		
DTaP-IPV-Hep B (Pediarix)	0.5 mL	IM
DTaP-IPB-Hib (Pentacel)		
DTaP-IPV (Kinrix; Quadracel)		
DTaP-IPV-Hib-HepB (Vaxelis)		
Hib-HepB (Comvax)		
Hib-MenCY (MenHibrix)		
MMRV (Proquad)	≤12 years: 0.5 mL	SC
HepA–HepB (Twinrix)	≥18 years: 1.0 mL	IM

ID, intradermal; IM, intramuscular; SC, subcutaneous.

Table 5 INJECTION SITE AND NEEDLE SIZE

Subcutaneous (SC) Injection—*use a 23- to 25-gauge needle. Choose the injection site that is appropriate for the person's age and body mass.*

Age	Needle Length	Injection Site
Infants 1 to 12 months	5/8"	Fatty tissue over anterolateral thigh muscle
Children 12 months and older, adolescents, and adults	5/8"	Fatty tissue over anterolateral thigh muscle or fatty tissues over triceps

Intramuscular (IM) Injection—*use a 22- to 25-gauge needle. Choose the injection site and needle length that is appropriate to the person's age and body mass.*

Age	Needle Length	Injection Site
Newborns (first 28 days)	5/8"	Anterolateral thigh muscle
Infants (1–12 months)	1"	Anterolateral thigh muscle
Toddlers (1–2 years)	1" to 1¼"	Anterolateral thigh muscle or
	5/8" to 1"	Deltoid muscle of arm
Children and teenagers (3–18 years)	5/8" to 1"	Deltoid muscle of arm
	1" to 1¼"	
Adults 19 years or older		
Female or male <130 lbs	5/8" to 1"	Deltoid muscle of arm
Female or male 130 to 152 lbs	1"	Deltoid muscle of arm
Female 153 to 200 lbs	1" to 1.5"	Deltoid muscle of arm
Male 130 to 260 lbs		
Female ≥200 lbs	1.5"	Deltoid muscle of arm
Male ≥260 lbs		

PART II

VACCINES THROUGHOUT THE LIFE CYCLE

2024 INFANT, CHILD, AND ADOLESCENT IMMUNIZATION SCHEDULES

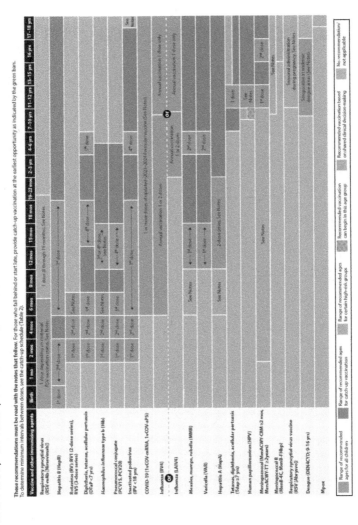

Figure 1 Recommended Child and Adolescent Immunization Schedule for Ages 18 Years or Younger, United States 2024. *Source: Centers for Disease Control and Prevention (www.cdc.gov).*

The table below provides catch-up schedules and minimum intervals between doses for children whose vaccinations have been delayed. A vaccine series does not need to be restarted, regardless of the time that has elapsed between doses. Use the section appropriate for the child's age. **Always use this table in conjunction with Table 1 and the Notes that follow.**

Vaccine	Minimum Age for Dose 1	Minimum Interval Between Doses			
		Dose 1 to Dose 2	Dose 2 to Dose 3	Dose 3 to Dose 4	Dose 4 to Dose 5
Children age 4 months through 6 years					
Hepatitis B	Birth	**4 weeks**	**8 weeks *and* at least 16 weeks after first dose** minimum age for the final dose is 24 weeks		
Rotavirus	6 weeks Maximum age for first dose is 14 weeks, 6 days.	**4 weeks**	**4 weeks** maximum age for final dose is 8 months, 0 days		
Diphtheria, tetanus, and acellular pertussis	6 weeks	**4 weeks**	**4 weeks**	**6 months**	**6 months** A fifth dose is not necessary if the fourth dose was administered at age 4 years or older **and** at least 6 months after dose 3
Haemophilus influenzae type b	6 weeks	**No further doses needed** if first dose was administered at age 15 months or older. **4 weeks** if first dose was administered before the 1st birthday. **8 weeks (as final dose)** if first dose was administered at age 12 through 14 months.	**No further doses needed** if previous dose was administered at age 15 months or older **4 weeks** if current age is younger than 12 months ***and*** first dose was administered at younger than age 7 months ***and*** at least 1 previous dose was PRP-T (ActHib®, Pentacel®, Hiberix®), Vaxelis® or unknown **8 weeks *and* age 12 through 59 months (as final dose)** if current age is younger than 12 months ***and*** first dose was administered at age 7 through 11 months; **OR** if current age is 12 through 59 months ***and*** first dose was administered before the 1st birthday ***and*** second dose was administered at younger than 15 months; **OR** if both doses were PedvaxHIB® and were administered before the 1st birthday	**8 weeks (as final dose)** This dose only necessary for children age 12 through 59 months who received 3 doses before the 1st birthday.	
Pneumococcal conjugate	6 weeks	**No further doses needed** for healthy children if first dose was administered at age 24 months or older **4 weeks** if first dose was administered before the 1st birthday **8 weeks (as final dose for healthy children)** if first dose was administered at the 1st birthday or after	**No further doses needed** for healthy children if previous dose was administered at age 24 months or older **4 weeks** if current age is younger than 12 months ***and*** previous dose was administered at <7 months old **8 weeks (as final dose for healthy children)** if previous dose was administered between 7–11 months (wait until at least 12 months old); **OR** if current age is 12 months or older ***and*** at least 1 dose was administered before age 12 months	**8 weeks (as final dose)** This dose is only necessary for children age 12 through 59 months regardless of risk, or age 60 through 71 months with any risk, who received 3 doses before age 12 months.	
Inactivated poliovirus	6 weeks	**4 weeks**	**4 weeks** if current age is <4 years **6 months (as final dose)** if current age is 4 years or older	**6 months (minimum age 4 years for final dose)**	
Measles, mumps, rubella	12 months	**4 weeks**			
Varicella	12 months	**3 months**			
Hepatitis A	12 months	**6 months**			
Meningococcal ACWY	2 months MenACWY-CRM 2 years MenACWY-TT	**8 weeks**	See Notes	See Notes	
Children and adolescents age 7 through 18 years					
Meningococcal ACWY	Not applicable (N/A)	**8 weeks**			
Tetanus, diphtheria; tetanus, diphtheria, and acellular pertussis	7 years	**4 weeks**	**4 weeks** if first dose of DTaP/DT was administered before the 1st birthday **6 months (as final dose)** if first dose of DTaP/DT or Tdap/Td was administered at or after the 1st birthday	**6 months** if first dose of DTaP/DT was administered before the 1st birthday	
Human papillomavirus	9 years	**Routine dosing intervals are recommended.**			
Hepatitis A	N/A	**6 months**			
Hepatitis B	N/A	**4 weeks**	**8 weeks *and* at least 16 weeks after first dose**		
Inactivated poliovirus	N/A	**4 weeks**	**6 months** A fourth dose is not necessary if the third dose was administered at age 4 years or older ***and*** at least 6 months after the previous dose.	A fourth dose of IPV is indicated if all previous doses were administered at <4 years **OR** if the third dose was administered <6 months after the second dose.	
Measles, mumps, rubella	N/A	**4 weeks**			
Varicella	N/A	**3 months** if younger than age 13 years. **4 weeks** if age 13 years or older			
Dengue	9 years	**6 months**	6 months		

Figure 2 Recommended Catch-up Immunization Schedule for Children and Adolescents Who Start Late or Who Are More Than 1 Month Behind, United States, 2024. *Source: Centers for Disease Control and Prevention (www.cdc.gov).*

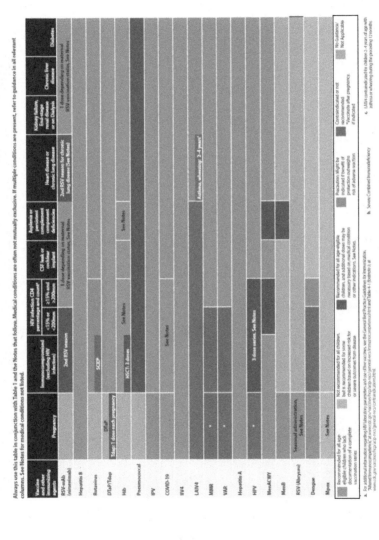

Figure 3 Recommended Child and Adolescent Immunization Schedule by Medical Indication, United States, 2024. *Source: Centers for Disease Control and Prevention (www.cdc.gov).*

Figure 4 Notes: Recommended Child and Adolescent Immunization Schedule for Ages 18 Years or Younger, United States, 2024. *Source: Centers for Disease Control and Prevention (www.cdc.gov).*

Notes Recommended Child and Adolescent Immunization Schedule for Ages 18 Years or Younger, United States, 2024

- **Previously vaccinated¹ with 3 or more doses of any Moderna or Pfizer-BioNTech:** 1 dose of updated (2023–2024 Formula) Moderna or Pfizer-BioNTech at least 8 weeks after the most recent dose.
- **Unvaccinated:**
  - 3-dose series of updated (2023–2024 Formula) Moderna at 0, 4, 8 weeks
  - 3-dose series of updated (2023–2024 Formula) Pfizer-BioNTech at 0, 3, 7 weeks
  - 2-dose series of updated (2023–2024 Formula) Novavax at 0, 3 weeks
- **Previously vaccinated¹ with 1 dose of any Moderna:** 2-dose series of updated (2023–2024 Formula) Moderna at 0, 4 weeks (minimum interval between previous Moderna dose and dose 1: 4 weeks).
- **Previously vaccinated¹ with 2 doses of any Moderna:** 1 dose of updated (2022–2024 Formula) Moderna at least 4 weeks after the most recent dose.
- **Previously vaccinated¹ with 1 dose of any Pfizer-BioNTech:** 2-dose series of updated (2023–2024 Formula) Pfizer-BioNTech at 0, 4 weeks (minimum interval between previous Pfizer-BioNTech dose and dose 1: 3 weeks).
- **Previously vaccinated¹ with 2 doses of any Pfizer-BioNTech:** 1 dose of updated (2023–2024 Formula) Pfizer-BioNTech at least 8 weeks after the most recent dose.
- **Previously vaccinated¹ with 3 or more doses of any Moderna or Pfizer-BioNTech:** 1 dose of any updated (2023–2024 Formula) COVID-19 vaccine at least 8 weeks after the most recent dose.
- **Previously vaccinated¹ with 1 or more doses of Janssen or Novavax or with or without dose(s) of any Original monovalent or bivalent COVID-19 vaccine:** 1 dose of any updated (2023–2024 Formula) COVID-19 vaccine at least 8 weeks after the most recent dose.

There is no preferential recommendation for the use of one COVID-19 vaccine over another when more than one age-appropriate vaccine is available.

Administer an age-appropriate COVID-19 vaccine product for each dose. For information about transition from age 4 years to age 5 years or age 11 years to age 12 years during COVID-19 vaccination series, see Tables 1 and 2 at www.cdc.gov/vaccines/covid-19/clinical-considerations/interim-considerations-us.html#covid-vaccines.

Current COVID-19 schedule and dosage formulation available at www.cdc.gov/covidschedule. For more information on Emergency Use Authorization (EUA) indications for COVID-19 vaccines, see www.fda.gov/emergency-preparedness-and-response/coronavirus-disease-2019-covid-19/covid-19-vaccines

¹**Note:** Previously vaccinated is defined as having received any Original monovalent or bivalent COVID-19 vaccine (Janssen, Moderna, Novavax, Pfizer-BioNTech) prior to the updated 2023–2024 formulation.

Note: Persons who are moderately or severely immunocompromised have the option to receive one additional dose of updated (2023–2024 Formula) COVID-19 vaccine at least 2 months following the last recommended updated (2023–2024 Formula) COVID-19 vaccine dose. Further additional doses of updated (2023–2024 Formula) COVID-19 vaccine dose(s) may be administered, informed by the clinical judgement of a healthcare provider and personal preference and circumstances. Any further additional doses should be administered at least 2 months after the last updated (2023–2024 Formula) COVID-19 vaccine dose. Moderately or severely immunocompromised children 6 months–4 years of age should receive homologous updated (2023–2024 Formula) mRNA vaccine dose(s) if they receive additional doses.

Dengue vaccination (minimum age: 9 years)

Routine vaccination
- Age 9–16 years living in areas with endemic dengue AND have laboratory confirmation of previous dengue infection
  - 3-dose series administered at 0, 6, and 12 months
- Endemic areas include Puerto Rico, Federated States of Micronesia, Republic of Marshall Islands, and the Republic of Palau. For updated guidance on testing see www.cdc.gov/mmwr/volumes/70/rr/rr7006a1.htm?s_cid=rr7006a1_w and www.cdc.gov/dengue/vaccine/hcp/index.html
- Dengue vaccine should not be administered to children travelling to or visiting endemic dengue areas.

Diphtheria, tetanus, and pertussis (DTaP) vaccination (minimum age: 6 weeks [4 years for Kinrix or Quadracel¹])

Routine vaccination
- 5-dose series (3-dose primary series at age 2, 4, and 6 months, followed by booster doses at ages 15–18 months and 4–6 years

- **Prospectively:** Dose 4 may be administered as early as age 12 months if at least 6 months have elapsed since dose 3.
- **Retrospectively:** A 4th dose that was inadvertently administered as early as age 12 months may be counted if at least 4 months have elapsed since dose 3.

Catch-up vaccination
- Dose 5 is not necessary if dose 4 was administered at age 4 years or older and at least 6 months after dose 3.
- For other catch-up guidance, see Table 2.

Special situations
- **Wound management** in children less than age 7 years with history of 3 or more doses of tetanus-toxoid-containing vaccine: For all wounds except clean and minor wounds, administer DTaP if more than 5 years since last dose of tetanus-toxoid-containing vaccine. For detailed information, see www.cdc.gov/mmwr/volumes/67/rr/rr6702a1.htm.

Haemophilus influenzae type b vaccination (minimum age: 6 weeks)

Routine vaccination
- **ActHIB®, Hiberix®, Pentacel®, or Vaxelis™:** 4-dose series (3-dose primary series at age 2, 4, and 6 months, followed by a booster dose* at age 12–15 months)
  - *Vaxelis™ is not recommended for use as a booster dose. A different Hib-containing vaccine should be used for the booster dose.
- **PedvaxHIB®:** 3-dose series (2-dose primary series at age 2 and 4 months, followed by a booster dose at age 12–15 months)

Catch-up vaccination
- **Dose 1 at age 7–11 months:** Administer dose 2 at least 4 weeks later and dose 3 (final dose) at age 12–15 months or 8 weeks after dose 2 (whichever is later).
- **Dose 1 at age 12–14 months:** Administer dose 2 (final dose) at least 8 weeks after dose 1.
- **Dose 1 before age 12 months and dose 2 before age 15 months:** Administer dose 3 (final dose) at least 8 weeks after dose 2.
- **2 doses of PedvaxHIB® before age 12 months:** Administer dose 3 (final dose) at age 12–59 months and at least 8 weeks after dose 2.
- **1 dose administered at age 15 months or older:** No further doses needed
- **Unvaccinated at age 15–59 months:** Administer 1 dose.

Figure 4 Continued

Notes — Recommended Child and Adolescent Immunization Schedule for Ages 18 Years or Younger, United States, 2024

- Previously unvaccinated children age 60 months or older who are not considered high risk: Do not require catch-up vaccination.

For other catch-up guidance, see Table 2. Vaxelis® can be used for catch-up vaccination in children less than age 5 years. Follow the catch-up schedule even if Vaxelis® is used for one or more doses. For detailed information on use of Vaxelis®, see www.cdc.gov/mmwr/volumes/69/wr/mm6905a5.htm.

Special situations

Chemotherapy or radiation treatment:
Age 12–59 months
- Unvaccinated or only 1 dose before age 12 months: 2 doses, 8 weeks apart
- 2 or more doses before age 12 months: 1 dose at least 8 weeks after previous dose

Doses administered within 14 days of starting therapy or during therapy should be repeated at least 3 months after therapy completion.

Hematopoietic stem cell transplant (HSCT):
- 3-dose series 4 weeks apart starting 6 to 12 months after successful transplant, regardless of Hib vaccination history

Anatomic or functional asplenia (including sickle cell disease):
Age 12–59 months
- Unvaccinated or only 1 dose before age 12 months: 2 doses, 8 weeks apart
- 2 or more doses before age 12 months: 1 dose at least 8 weeks after previous dose
Unvaccinated* persons age 5 years or older
- 1 dose

Elective splenectomy:
Unvaccinated* persons age 15 months or older
- 1 dose (preferably at least 14 days before procedure)

HIV infection:
Age 12–59 months
- Unvaccinated or only 1 dose before age 12 months: 2 doses, 8 weeks apart
- 2 or more doses before age 12 months: 1 dose at least 8 weeks after previous dose
Unvaccinated* persons age 5–18 years
- 1 dose

Immunoglobulin deficiency, early component complement deficiency:
Age 12–59 months
- Unvaccinated or only 1 dose before age 12 months: 2 doses, 8 weeks apart

- 2 or more doses before age 12 months: 1 dose at least 8 weeks after previous dose

*Unvaccinated = Less than routine series (through age 14 months) OR no doses (age 15 months or older)

Hepatitis A vaccination
(minimum age: 12 months for routine vaccination)

Routine vaccination
- 2-dose series (minimum interval: 6 months) at age 12–23 months

Catch-up vaccination
- Unvaccinated persons through age 18 years should complete a 2-dose series (minimum interval: 6 months).
- Persons who previously received 1 dose at age 12 months or older should receive dose 2 at least 6 months after dose 1.
- Adolescents age 18 years or older may receive the combined HepA and HepB vaccine, Twinrix®, as a 3-dose series (0, 1, and 6 months) or 4-dose series (3 doses at 0, 7, and 21–30 days, followed by a booster dose at 12 months).

International travel
- Persons traveling to or working in countries with high or intermediate endemic hepatitis A (www.cdc.gov/travel/):
- Infants age 6–11 months: 1 dose before departure; revaccinate with 2 doses (separated by at least 6 months) between age 12–23 months.
- Unvaccinated age 12 months or older. Administer dose 1 as soon as travel is considered.

Hepatitis B vaccination
(minimum age: birth)

Routine vaccination
- 3-dose series at age 0, 1–2, 6–18 months (use monovalent HepB vaccine for doses administered before age 6 weeks)
- Birth weight ≥2,000 grams: 1 dose within 24 hours of birth if medically stable
- Birth weight <2,000 grams: 1 dose at chronological age 1 month or hospital discharge (whichever is earlier and even if weight is still <2,000 grams).
- Infants who did not receive a birth dose should begin the series as soon as possible (see Table 2 for minimum intervals).
- Administration of 4 doses is permitted when a combination vaccine containing HepB is used after the birth dose.
- Minimum intervals (see Table 2): when 4 doses are administered, substitute "dose 4" for "dose 3" in these calculations

- Final (3rd or 4th) dose: age 6–18 months (minimum age 24 weeks)

Mother is HBsAg-positive
- Birth dose (monovalent HepB vaccine only): administer HepB vaccine and hepatitis B immune globulin (HBIG) (in separate limbs) within 12 hours of birth, regardless of birth weight.
- Birth weight <2,000 grams: administer 3 additional doses of HepB vaccine beginning at age 1 month (total of 4 doses)
- Final (3rd or 4th) dose: administer at age 6 months (minimum age 24 weeks)
- Test for HBsAg and anti-HBs at age 9–12 months. If HepB series is delayed, test 1–2 months after final dose. Do not test before age 9 months.

Mother is HBsAg-unknown
- If other evidence suggestive of maternal hepatitis B infection exists (e.g., presence of HBV DNA, HBsAg-positive, or mother known to have chronic hepatitis B infection), manage infant as if mother is HBsAg-positive
- Birth dose (monovalent HepB vaccine only):
- Birth weight ≥2,000 grams: administer HepB vaccine within 12 hours of birth. Determine mother's HBsAg-positive, administer HBIG as soon as possible (in separate limbs), but no later than 7 days of age.
- Birth weight <2,000 grams: administer HepB vaccine and HBIG (in separate limbs) within 12 hours of birth. Administer 3 additional doses of HepB vaccine beginning at age 1 month (total of 4 doses)
- Final (3rd or 4th) dose: administer at age 6 months (minimum age 24 weeks)
- If mother is determined to be HBsAg-positive or if status remains unknown, test for HBsAg and anti-HBs at age 9–12 months. If HepB series is delayed, test 1–2 months after final dose. Do not test before age 9 months.

Catch-up vaccination
- Unvaccinated persons should complete a 3-dose series at 0, 1–2, 6 months. See Table 2 for minimum intervals
- Adolescents age 11–15 years may use an alternative 2-dose schedule with at least 4 months between doses (adult formulation Recombivax HB®) only.
- Adolescents age 18 years may receive:
- Heplisav-B® : 2-dose series at least 4 weeks apart
- PreHevbrio® : 3-dose series at 0, 1, and 6 months
- Combined HepA and HepB vaccine, Twinrix® : 3-dose series (0, 1, and 6 months) or 4-dose series (3 doses at 0, 7, and 21–30 days, followed by a booster dose at 12 months).

Figure 4 Continued

Notes Recommended Child and Adolescent Immunization Schedule for Ages 18 Years or Younger, United States, 2024

Special situations
- Revaccination is not generally recommended for persons with a normal immune status who were vaccinated as infants, children, adolescents, or adults.
- Post-vaccination serology testing and revaccination (if anti-HBs <10mIU/mL) is recommended for certain populations, including:
  - Infants born to HBsAg-positive mothers
  - Persons who are predialysis or on maintenance dialysis
  - Other immunocompromised persons
  - For detailed revaccination recommendations, see www.cdc. gov/vaccines/hcp/acip-recs/vacc-specific/hepb.html.

Note: Heplisav-B and PreHevbrio are not recommended in pregnancy due to lack of safety data in pregnant persons

Human papillomavirus vaccination
(minimum age: 9 years)

Routine and catch-up vaccination
- HPV vaccination routinely recommended at age 11–12 years (can start at age 9 years) and catch-up HPV vaccination recommended for all persons through age 18 years if not adequately vaccinated.
- 2- or 3-dose series depending on age at initial vaccination:
  - Age 9–14 years at initial vaccination: 2-dose series at 0, 6–12 months (minimum interval: 5 months; repeat dose if administered too soon)
  - Age 15 years or older at initial vaccination: 3-dose series at 0, 1–2 months, 6 months (minimum intervals: dose 1 to dose 2: 4 weeks / dose 2 to dose 3: 12 weeks / dose 1 to dose 3: 5 months; repeat dose if administered too soon)
- No additional dose recommended when any HPV vaccine series of any valency has been completed using recommended dosing intervals.

Special situations
- Immunocompromising conditions, including HIV infection: 3-dose series, even for those who initiate vaccination at age 9 through 14 years.
- History of sexual abuse or assault: Start at age 9 years
- Pregnancy: Pregnancy testing not needed before vaccination; HPV vaccination not recommended until after pregnancy; no intervention needed if vaccinated while pregnant

Influenza vaccination
(minimum age: 6 months [IIV], 2 years [LAIV4], 18 years [recombinant influenza vaccine, RIV4])

Routine vaccination
- Use any influenza vaccine appropriate for age and health status annually:
  - Age 6 months–8 years who have received fewer than 2 influenza vaccine doses before July 1, 2023, or whose influenza vaccination history is unknown: 2 doses, separated by at least 4 weeks. Administer dose 2 even if the child turns 9 years between receipt of dose 1 and dose 2.
  - Age 6 months–8 years who have received at least 2 influenza vaccine doses before July 1, 2023: 1 dose
  - Age 9 years or older: 1 dose
- For the 2023–2024 season, see www.cdc.gov/mmwr/volumes/72/rr/rr7202a1.htm.
- For the 2024–25 season, see the 2024–25 ACIP influenza vaccine recommendations.

Special situations
- Close contacts (e.g., household contacts) of severely immunosuppressed persons who require a protected environment should not receive LAIV4. If LAIV4 is given, they should avoid contact with for such immunosuppressed persons for 7 days after vaccination.
- Note: Persons with an egg allergy can receive any influenza vaccine (egg-based and non-egg-based) appropriate for age and health status.

Measles, mumps, and rubella vaccination
(minimum age: 12 months for routine vaccination)

Routine vaccination
- 2-dose series at age 12–15 months, age 4–6 years
- MMR or MMRV may be administered
- Note: For dose 1 in children age 12–47 months, it is recommended to administer MMR and varicella vaccines separately. MMRV may be used if parents or caregivers express a preference.

Catch-up vaccination
- Unvaccinated children and adolescents: 2-dose series at least 4 weeks apart*
- The maximum age for use of MMRV is 12 years.

Special situations
- International travel
  - Infants age 6–11 months: 1 dose before departure; revaccinate with 2-dose series at age 12–15 months (12 months for children in high-risk areas) and dose 2 as early as 4 weeks later.*
  - Unvaccinated children age 12 months or older: 2-dose series at least 4 weeks apart before departure*
- In mumps outbreak settings, for information about additional doses of MMR (including 3rd dose of MMR), see www.cdc.gov/mmwr/volumes/67/wr/mm6701a7.htm

*Note: If MMRV is used, the minimum interval between MMRV doses is 3 months

Meningococcal serogroup A,C,W,Y vaccination
(minimum age: 2 months [MenACWY-CRM, Menveo], 2 years [MenACWY-TT, MenQuadfi]), 10 years [MenACWY-TT/MenB-FHbp, Penbraya])

Routine vaccination
- 2-dose series at age 11–12 years; 16 years

Catch-up vaccination
- Age 13–15 years: 1 dose now and booster at age 16–18 years (minimum interval: 8 weeks)
- Age 16–18 years: 1 dose

Special situations
Anatomic or functional asplenia (including sickle cell disease), HIV infection, persistent complement component deficiency, complement inhibitor (e.g., eculizumab, ravulizumab) use:
- **Menveo**
  - Dose 1 at age 2 months: 4-dose series (additional 3 doses at age 4, 6, and 12 months)
  - Dose 1 at age 3–6 months: 3- or 4-dose series (dose 2 [and dose 3 if applicable] at least 8 weeks after previous dose until a dose is received at age 7 months or older, followed by an additional dose at least 12 weeks later and after age 12 months)
  - Dose 1 at age 7–23 months: 2-dose series (dose 2 at least 12 weeks after dose 1 and after age 12 months)
  - Dose 1 at age 24 months or older: 2-dose series at least 8 weeks apart
- **MenQuadfi**
  - Dose 1 at age 24 months or older: 2-dose series at least 8 weeks apart

Figure 4 Continued

Notes — Recommended Child and Adolescent Immunization Schedule for Ages 18 Years or Younger, United States, 2024

Travel to countries with hyperendemic or epidemic meningococcal disease, including countries in the African meningitis belt or during the Hajj (www.cdc.gov/travel/):
- Children less than age 24 months:
  - Menveo® (age 2–23 months):
    - Dose 1 at age 2 months: 4-dose series (additional 3 doses at age 4, 6, and 12 months)
    - Dose 1 at age 3–6 months: 3- or 4-dose series (dose 2 [and dose 3 if applicable] at least 8 weeks after previous dose until a dose is received at age 7 months or older, followed by an additional dose at least 12 weeks later and age 12 months)
    - Dose 1 at age 7–23 months: 2-dose series (dose 2 at least 12 weeks after dose 1 and after age 12 months)
  - Children age 2 years or older: 1 dose Menveo® or MenQuadfi®

First-year college students who live in residential housing (if not previously vaccinated at age 16 years or older) or military recruits:
- 1 dose Menveo® or MenQuadfi®

Adolescent vaccination of children who received MenACWY prior to age 10 years:
- Children for whom boosters are recommended because of an ongoing increased risk of meningococcal disease (e.g., those with complement component deficiency, HIV, or asplenia): Follow the booster schedule for persons at increased risk.
- Children for whom boosters are not recommended (e.g., a healthy child who received a single dose for travel to a country where meningococcal disease is endemic): Administer MenACWY according to the recommended adolescent schedule with dose 1 at age 11–12 years and dose 2 at age 16 years.

Menveo has two formulations: lyophilized and liquid. The liquid formulation should not be used before age 10 years. See www.cdc.gov/vaccines/vpd/mening/downloads/menveo-single-vial-presentation.pdf.

Note: For MenACWY booster dose recommendations for groups listed under "Special situations" and in an outbreak setting and additional meningococcal vaccination information, see www.cdc.gov/mmwr/volumes/69/rr/rr6909a1.htm.

Children age 10 years or older may receive a single dose of Penbraya™ as an alternative to separate administration of MenACWY and MenB when both vaccines would be given on the same clinic day (see "Meningococcal serogroup B vaccination" section below for more information).

Meningococcal serogroup B vaccination
(minimum age: 10 years [MenB-4C, Bexsero®; MenB-FHbp, Trumenba®; MenACWY-TT/MenB-FHbp, Penbraya™])

Shared clinical decision-making
- Adolescents not at increased risk age 16–23 years (preferred age 16–18 years) based on shared clinical decision-making:
  - Bexsero®: 2-dose series at least 1 month apart
  - Trumenba®: 2-dose series at least 6 months apart (if dose 2 is administered earlier than 6 months, administer 3rd dose at least 4 months after dose 2)

For additional information on shared clinical decision-making for MenB, see www.cdc.gov/vaccines/hcp/admin/downloads/isd-job-aid-scdm-mening-b-shared-clinical-decision-making.pdf

Special situations
Anatomic or functional asplenia (including sickle cell disease), persistent complement component deficiency, complement inhibitor (e.g., eculizumab, ravulizumab) use:
- Bexsero®: 2-dose series at least 1 month apart
- Trumenba®: 3-dose series at 0, 1–2, 6 months (if dose 2 was administered at least 6 months after dose 1, dose 3 not needed; if dose 3 is administered earlier than 4 months after dose 2, a 4th dose should be administered at least 4 months after dose 3)

Note: Bexsero® and Trumenba® are not interchangeable; the same product should be used for all doses in a series.

For MenB booster dose recommendations for groups listed under "Special situations" and in an outbreak setting and additional meningococcal vaccination information, see www.cdc.gov/mmwr/volumes/69/rr/rr6909a3.htm.

Children age 10 years or older may receive a dose of Penbraya™ as an alternative to separate administration of MenACWY and MenB when both vaccines would be given on the same clinic day. For age-eligible children not at increased risk, if Penbraya™ is used for dose 1 MenB, MenB-FHbp (Trumenba) should be administered for dose 2 MenB. For age-eligible children at increased risk of meningococcal disease, Penbraya™ may be used for additional MenACWY and MenB doses (including booster doses) if both would be given on the same clinic day and at least 6 months have elapsed since most recent Penbraya™ dose.

Mpox vaccination
(minimum age: 18 years [Jynneos®])

Special situations
- Age 18 years and at risk for Mpox infection: 2-dose series, 28 days apart.
- Risk factors for Mpox infection include:
  - Persons who are gay, bisexual, and other MSM, transgender or nonbinary people who in the past 6 months have had:
    - A new diagnosis of at least 1 sexually transmitted disease
    - More than 1 sex partner
    - Sex at a commercial sex venue
    - Sex in association with a large public event in a geographic area where Mpox transmission is occurring
  - Persons who are sexual partners of the persons described above
  - Persons who anticipate experiencing any of the situations described above
- Pregnancy: There is currently no ACIP recommendation for Jynneos use in pregnancy due to lack of safety data in pregnant persons. Pregnant persons with any risk factor described above may receive Jynneos.

For detailed information, see www.cdc.gov/vaccines/acip/meetings/downloads/slides-2023-10-25-26/04-MPOX-Rao-508.pdf

---

Pneumococcal vaccination
(minimum age: 6 weeks [PCV15], PCV20; 2 years [PPSV23])

Routine vaccination with PCV
- 4-dose series at 2, 4, 6, 12–15 months

Catch-up vaccination with PCV
- Healthy children ages 2–4 years with any incomplete* PCV series: 1 dose PCV
- For other catch-up guidance, see Table 2.

Note: For children without risk conditions, PCV20 is not indicated if they have received 4 doses of PCV13 or PCV15 or another age-appropriate complete PCV series.

Figure 4 Continued

Notes

Recommended Child and Adolescent Immunization Schedule for Ages 18 Years or Younger, United States, 2024

Special situations

Children and adolescents with cerebrospinal fluid leak; chronic heart disease; chronic kidney disease (excluding maintenance dialysis and nephrotic syndrome); chronic liver disease; chronic lung disease (including moderate persistent or severe persistent asthma); cochlear implant; or diabetes mellitus:

Age 2–5 years
- Any incomplete* PCV series with:
  - 3 PCV doses: 1 dose PCV (at least 8 weeks after the most recent PCV dose
  - Less than 3 PCV doses: 2 doses PCV (at least 8 weeks after the most recent dose and administered at least 8 weeks apart)
- Completed recommended PCV series but have not received PPSV23
  - Previously received at least 1 dose of PCV20: no further PCV or PPSV23 doses needed
  - Not previously received PCV20: administer 1 dose PCV20 OR 1 dose PPSV23 at least 8 weeks after the most recent PCV dose. If PPSV23 is used, administer 1 dose of PCV20 or dose 2 PPSV23 at least 5 years after dose 1 PPSV23.

Age 6–18 years
- Not previously received any dose of PCV13, PCV15, or PCV20: administer 1 dose of PCV15 or 1 dose of PCV20. If PCV15 is used and no previous receipt of PPSV23, administer 1 dose of PPSV23 at least 8 weeks after the PCV15 dose.**
- Received PCV before age 6 years but have not received PPSV23
  - Previously received at least 1 dose of PCV20: no further PCV or PPSV23 doses needed
  - Not previously received PCV20: administer 1 dose PCV20 OR 1 dose PPSV23 at least 8 weeks after the most recent PCV dose.**

Children and adolescents on maintenance dialysis, or with immunocompromising conditions such as nephrotic syndrome; congenital or acquired asplenia or splenic dysfunction; congenital or acquired immunodeficiencies; diseases and conditions treated with immunosuppressive drugs or radiation therapy, including malignant neoplasms, leukemias, lymphomas, Hodgkin disease, and solid organ transplant; HIV infection; or sickle cell disease or other hemoglobinopathies:

Age 2–5 years
- Any incomplete* PCV series:
  - 3 PCV doses: 1 dose PCV (at least 8 weeks after the most recent PCV dose)
  - Less than 3 PCV doses: 2 doses PCV (at least 8 weeks after the most recent dose and administered at least 8 weeks apart)
- Completed recommended PCV series but have not received PPSV23
  - Previously received at least 1 dose of PCV20: no further PCV or PPSV23 doses needed
  - Not previously received PCV20: administer 1 dose PCV20 OR 1 dose PPSV23 at least 8 weeks after the most recent PCV dose. If PPSV23 is used, administer 1 dose of PCV20 or dose 2 PPSV23 at least 5 years after dose 1 PPSV23.

Age 6–18 years
- Not previously received any dose of PCV13, PCV15, or PCV20: administer 1 dose of PCV15 or PCV20. If PCV15 is used and no previous receipt of PPSV23, administer either PCV20 or dose 2 PPSV23 at least 5 years after dose 1 PPSV23.
- Received PCV13 only at or after age 6 years: administer 1 dose PCV20 OR 1 dose PPSV23 at least 8 weeks after the most recent PCV13 dose. If PPSV23 is used, administer 1 dose of PCV20 or dose 2 PPSV23 at least 5 years after dose 1 PPSV23
- Received 1 dose PCV13 and 1 dose PPSV23 at or after age 6 years: administer 1 dose PCV20 OR 1 dose PPSV23 at least 8 weeks after the most recent PCV13 dose and at least 5 years after dose 1 PPSV23.
- *Incomplete series = Not having received all doses in either the recommended series or an age-appropriate catch-up series. See Table 2 in ACIP pneumococcal recommendations at stacks.cdc.gov/view/cdc/133252
- **When both PCV15 and PPSV23 are indicated, administer all doses of PCV15 first. PCV15 and PPSV23 should not be administered during the same visit.

For guidance on determining which pneumococcal vaccines a patient needs and when, please refer to the mobile app, which can be downloaded here: www.cdc.gov/vaccines/vpd/pneumo/hcp/pneumoapp.html

Poliovirus vaccination
(minimum age: 6 weeks)

Routine vaccination
- 4-dose series at ages 2, 4, 6–18 months, 4–6 years; administer the final dose on or after age 4 years and at least 6 months after the previous dose.
- 4 or more doses of IPV can be administered before age 4 years when a combination vaccine containing IPV is used. However, a dose is still recommended on or after age 4 years and at least 6 months after the previous dose.

Catch-up vaccination
- In the first 6 months of life, use minimum ages and intervals only for travel to a polio-endemic region or during an outbreak.
- Adolescents age 18 years known or suspected to be unvaccinated or incompletely vaccinated: administer remaining doses (1, 2, or 3 IPV doses) to complete a 3-dose primary series.* Unless there are specific reasons to believe they were not vaccinated, most persons aged 18 years or older born and raised in the United States can assume they were vaccinated against polio as children.

Series containing oral poliovirus vaccine (OPV), either mixed OPV-IPV or OPV-only series:
- Total number of doses needed to complete the series is the same as that recommended for the U.S. IPV schedule. See www.cdc.gov/mmwr/volumes/66/wr/mm6601a6.htm?s_%20cid=mm6601a6_w.
- Only trivalent OPV (tOPV) counts toward the U.S. vaccination requirements.
  - Doses of OPV administered before April 1, 2016, should be counted (unless specifically noted as administered during a campaign).
  - Doses of OPV administered on or after April 1, 2016, should not be counted.
- For guidance to assess doses documented as "OPV," see www.cdc.gov/mmwr/volumes/66/wr/mm6606a7.htm?s_cid=mm6606a7_w.
- For catch-up guidance, see Table 2.

Figure 4 Continued

Notes Recommended Child and Adolescent Immunization Schedule for Ages 18 Years or Younger, United States, 2024

Special situations
- Adolescents aged 18 years at increased risk of exposure to poliovirus and completed primary series*: may administer one lifetime IPV booster

*Note: Complete primary series consist of at least 3 doses of IPV or trivalent oral poliovirus vaccine (tOPV) in any combination.

For detailed information, see: www.cdc.gov/vaccines/vpd/polio/hcp/recommendations.html

Respiratory syncytial virus immunization
(minimum age: birth [Nirsevimab, RSV-mAb (Beyfortus™)])

Routine immunization
- **Infants born October – March in most of the continental United States***
  - Mother did not receive RSV vaccine OR mother's RSV vaccination status is unknown: administer 1 dose nirsevimab within 1 week of birth in hospital or outpatient setting
  - Mother received RSV vaccine less than 14 days prior to delivery: administer 1 dose nirsevimab within 1 week of birth in hospital or outpatient setting
  - Mother received RSV vaccine at least 14 days prior to delivery: nirsevimab not needed but can be considered in rare circumstances at the discretion of healthcare providers (see special populations and situations at www.cdc.gov/vaccines/vpd/rsv/hcp/child-faqs.html)
- **Infants born April–September in most of the continental United States***
  - Mother did not receive RSV vaccine OR mother's RSV vaccination status is unknown: administer 1 dose nirsevimab shortly before start of RSV season*
  - Mother received RSV vaccine less than 14 days prior to delivery: administer 1 dose nirsevimab shortly before start of RSV season*
  - Mother received RSV vaccine at least 14 days prior to delivery: nirsevimab not needed but can be considered in rare circumstances at the discretion of healthcare providers/special populations and situations at www.cdc.gov/vaccines/vpd/rsv/hcp/child-faqs.html

Infants with prolonged birth hospitalization** (e.g., for prematurity) discharged October through March should be immunized shortly before or promptly after discharge.

Special situations
- **Ages 8–19 months with chronic lung disease of prematurity requiring medical support (e.g., chronic corticosteroid therapy, diuretic therapy, or supplemental oxygen) any time during the 6-month period before the start of the second RSV season; severe immunocompromise; cystic fibrosis with either weight for length <10th percentile or manifestation of severe lung disease (e.g., previous hospitalization for pulmonary exacerbation in the first year of life or abnormalities on chest imaging that persist when stable)**:**
  - 1 dose nirsevimab shortly before start of second RSV season*
- **Ages 8–19 months who are American Indian or Alaska Native:**
  - 1 dose nirsevimab shortly before start of second RSV season*
- Age-eligible and undergoing cardiac surgery with cardiopulmonary bypass**: 1 additional dose of nirsevimab after surgery. For additional details see special populations and situations at www.cdc.gov/vaccines/vpd/rsv/hcp/child-faqs.html

*Note: While the timing of the onset and duration of RSV season may vary, nirsevimab may be administered October through March in most of the continental United States. Providers in jurisdictions with RSV seasonality that differs from most of the continental United States (e.g., Alaska, jurisdiction with tropical climate) should follow guidance from public health authorities (e.g., CDC, health departments) or regional medical centers on timing of administration based on local RSV seasonality. Although optimal timing of administration is just before the start of the RSV season, nirsevimab may also be administered during the RSV season to infants and children who are age-eligible.

**Nirsevimab can be administered to children who are eligible to receive palivizumab. Children who have received nirsevimab should not receive palivizumab for the same RSV season.

For further guidance, see www.cdc.gov/mmwr/volumes/72/wr/mm7234a4.htm and www.cdc.gov/vaccines/vpd/rsv/hcp/child-faqs.html

Respiratory syncytial virus vaccination (RSV [Abrysvo™])

Routine vaccination
- Pregnant at 32 weeks 0 days through 36 weeks and 6 days gestation from September through January in most of the continental United States†: 1 dose RSV vaccine (Abrysvo™). Administer RSV vaccine regardless of previous RSV infection.
- Either maternal RSV vaccination or infant immunization with nirsevimab (RSV monoclonal antibody) is recommended to prevent respiratory syncytial virus lower respiratory tract infection in infants.

- All other pregnant persons: RSV vaccine not recommended. There is currently no ACIP recommendation for RSV vaccination in subsequent pregnancies. No data are available to inform whether additional doses are needed in later pregnancies.

†Note: Providers in jurisdictions with RSV seasonality differs from most of the continental United States (e.g., Alaska, jurisdiction with tropical climate) should follow guidance from public health authorities (e.g., CDC, health departments) or regional medical centers on timing of administration based on local RSV seasonality.

Rotavirus vaccination
(minimum age: 6 weeks)

Routine vaccination
- **Rotarix®**: 2-dose series at age 2 and 4 months
- **RotaTeq®**: 3-dose series at age 2, 4, and 6 months
- If any dose in the series is either **RotaTeq®** or unknown, default to 3-dose series.

Catch-up vaccination
- Do not start the series on or after age 15 weeks, 0 days.
- The maximum age for the final dose is 8 months, 0 days.
- For other catch-up guidance, see Table 2.

Figure 4 Continued

Notes

Recommended Child and Adolescent Immunization Schedule for Ages 18 Years or Younger, United States, 2024

Tetanus, diphtheria, and pertussis (Tdap) vaccination
(minimum age: 11 years for routine vaccination, 7 years for catch-up vaccination)

Routine vaccination
- **Age 11–12 years:** 1 dose Tdap (adolescent booster)
- **Pregnancy:** 1 dose Tdap during each pregnancy, preferably in early part of gestational weeks 27–36.

Note: Tdap may be administered regardless of the interval since the last tetanus- and diphtheria-toxoid-containing vaccine.

Catch-up vaccination
- **Age 13–18 years who have not received Tdap:** 1 dose Tdap (adolescent booster)
- **Age 7–18 years not fully vaccinated* with DTaP:** 1 dose Tdap as part of the catch-up series (preferably the first dose); if additional doses are needed, use Td or Tdap.
  - **Tdap administered at age 7–10 years:**
    - **Age 7–9 years** who receive Tdap should receive the adolescent Tdap booster dose at age 11–12 years.
    - **Age 10 years** who receive Tdap do not need the adolescent Tdap booster dose at age 11–12 years.
  - **DTaP inadvertently administered on or after age 7 years:**
    - **Age 7–9 years:** DTaP may count as part of catch-up series. Administer adolescent Tdap booster dose at age 11–12 years.
    - **Age 10–18 years:** Count dose of DTaP as the adolescent Tdap booster dose.
- For other catch-up guidance, see Table 2.

Special situations
- **Wound management** in persons age 7 years or older with history of 3 or more doses of tetanus-toxoid-containing vaccine: For clean and minor wounds, administer Tdap or Td if more than 10 years since last dose of tetanus-toxoid-containing vaccine; for all other wounds, administer Tdap or Td if more than 5 years since last dose of tetanus-toxoid-containing vaccine. Tdap is preferred for persons age 11 years or older who have not previously received Tdap or whose Tdap history is unknown. If a tetanus-toxoid-containing vaccine is indicated for a pregnant adolescent, use Tdap.
- For detailed information, see www.cdc.gov/mmwr/volumes/69/wr/mm6903a5.htm.

*Fully vaccinated = 5 valid doses of DTaP OR 4 valid doses of DTaP if dose 4 was administered at age 4 years or older

Varicella vaccination
(minimum age: 12 months)

Routine vaccination
- 2-dose series at age 12–15 months, 4–6 years
- VAR or MMRV may be administered*
- Dose 2 may be administered as early as 3 months after dose 1 (a dose inadvertently administered after at least 4 weeks may be counted as valid)

*Note: For dose 1 in children age 12–47 months, it is recommended to administer MMR and varicella vaccines separately. MMRV may be used if parents or caregivers express a preference.

Catch-up vaccination
- Ensure persons age 7–18 years without evidence of immunity (see MMWR at www.cdc.gov/mmwr/pdf/rr/rr5604.pdf) have a 2-dose series:
  - **Age 7–12 years:** Routine interval: 3 months (a dose inadvertently administered after at least 4 weeks may be counted as valid)
  - **Age 13 years and older:** Routine interval: 4–8 weeks (minimum interval: 4 weeks)
  - The maximum age for use of MMRV is 12 years.

Figure 4 Continued

2024 ADULT IMMUNIZATION SCHEDULES

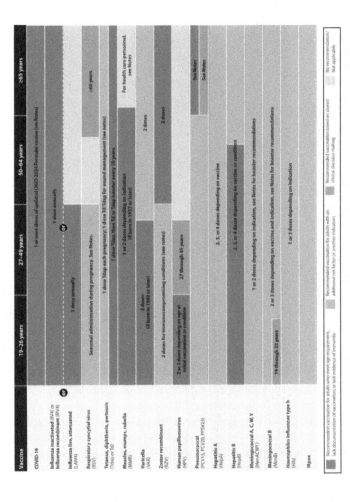

Figure 5 Recommended Adult Immunization Schedule by Age Group, United States, 2024. Source: *Centers for Disease Control and Prevention (www.cdc.gov)*.

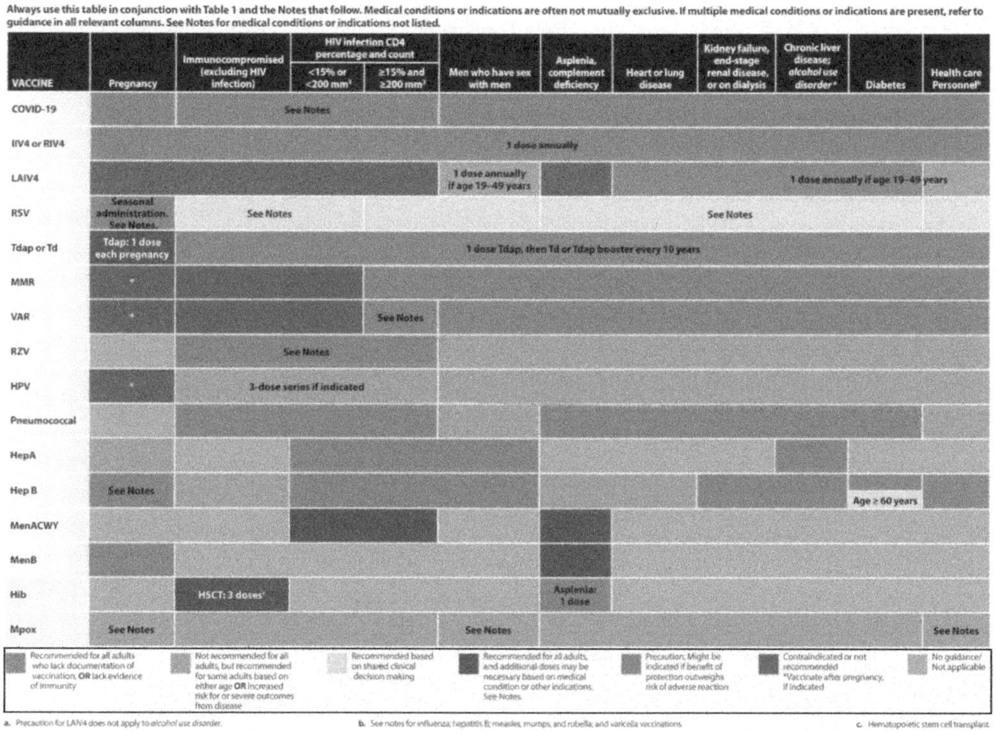

Figure 6 Recommended Adult Immunization Schedule by Medical Condition or Other Indication, United States, 2024. *Source: Centers for Disease Control and Prevention (www.cdc.gov).*

Notes Recommended Adult Immunization Schedule for Ages 19 Years or Older, United States, 2024

	COVID-19 vaccination	• Previously vaccinated* with 3 or more doses of any Moderna or Pfizer-BioNTech: 1 dose of any updated (2023–2024 Formula) COVID-19 vaccine at least 8 weeks after the most recent dose.
For vaccination recommendations for persons ages 18 years or younger, see the Recommended Child and Adolescent Immunization Schedule, 2024; www.cdc.gov/vaccines/schedules/hcp/child-adolescent.html	Routine vaccination Age 19 years or older	
Additional Information	• Unvaccinated: – 1 dose of updated (2023–2024 Formula) Moderna or Pfizer-BioNTech vaccine – 2-dose series of updated (2022–2024 Formula) Novavax at 0, 3–8 weeks	• Previously vaccinated* with 1 or more doses of Janssen or Novavax with or without dose(s) of any Original monovalent or bivalent COVID-19 vaccine: 1 dose of any updated (2023–2024 Formula) of COVID-19 vaccine at least 8 weeks after the most recent dose.
• For calculating intervals between doses, 4 weeks = 28 days, intervals of ≥4 months are determined by calendar months.		
• Within a number range (e.g., 12–18), a dash (–) should be read as "through."	• Previously vaccinated* with 1 or more doses of any COVID-19 vaccine: 1 dose of any updated (2023–2024 Formula) COVID-19 vaccine administered at least 8 weeks after the most recent COVID-19 vaccine dose.	There is no preferential recommendation for the use of one COVID-19 vaccine over another when more than one recommended age-appropriate vaccine is available.
• Vaccine doses administered ≤4 days before the minimum age or interval are considered valid. Doses of any vaccine administered ≥5 days earlier than the minimum age or minimum interval should not be counted as valid and should be repeated. **The repeat dose should be spaced after the invalid dose by the recommended minimum interval.** For further details, see Table 3-2, Recommended and minimum ages and intervals between vaccine doses, in *General Best Practice Guidelines for Immunization* at www.cdc.gov/vaccines/hcp/acip-recs/general-recs/timing.html.	Special situations Persons who are moderately or severely immunocompromised**	Current COVID-19 vaccine information available at www.cdc.gov/covidschedule. For information on Emergency Use Authorization (EUA) indications for COVID-19 vaccines, see www.fda.gov/emergency-preparedness-and-response/coronavirus-disease-2019-covid-19/covid-19-vaccines.
	• Unvaccinated: – 3-dose series of updated (2023–2024 Formula) Moderna at 0, 4, 8 weeks – 3-dose series of updated (2023–2024 Formula) Pfizer-BioNTech at 0, 3, 7 weeks – 2-dose series of updated (2023–2024 Formula) Novavax at 0, 3 weeks	*Note: Previously vaccinated is defined as having received any Original monovalent or bivalent COVID-19 vaccine (Janssen, Moderna, Novavax, Pfizer-BioNTech) prior to the updated 2023-2024 formulation.
• Information on travel vaccination requirements and recommendations is available at www.cdc.gov/travel/.		**Note: Persons who are moderately or severely immunocompromised may have the option to receive one additional dose of updated (2023-2024 Formula) COVID-19 vaccine at least 2 months following the last recommended (updated 2023-2024 Formula) COVID-19 vaccine dose. Further additional updated (2023-2024 Formula) COVID-19 vaccine dose(s) may be administered, informed by the clinical judgement of a healthcare provider and personal preference and circumstances. Any further additional doses should be administered at least 2 months after the last updated (2023-2024 Formula) COVID-19 vaccine dose.
• For vaccination of persons with immunodeficiencies, see Table 8-1, Vaccination of persons with primary and secondary immunodeficiencies, in *General Best Practice Guidelines for Immunization* at www.cdc.gov/vaccines/hcp/acip-recs/general-recs/immunocompetence.html	• Previously vaccinated* with 1 dose of any Moderna: 2-dose series of updated (2023–2024 Formula) Moderna at 0, 4 weeks (minimum interval between previous Moderna dose and dose 1-4 weeks)	
• For information about vaccination in the setting of a vaccine-preventable disease outbreak, contact your state or local health department.	• Previously vaccinated* with 2 doses of any Moderna: 1 dose of updated (2023–2024 Formula) Moderna at least 4 weeks after most recent dose.	
• The National Vaccine Injury Compensation Program (VICP) is a no-fault alternative to the traditional legal system for resolving vaccine injury claims. All vaccines included in the adult immunization schedule except PPSV23, RSV, RZV, Mpox, and COVID-19 vaccines are covered by the National Vaccine Injury Compensation Program (VICP). Mpox and COVID-19 vaccines are covered by the Countermeasures Injury Compensation Program (CICP). For more information, see www.hrsa.gov/vaccinecompensation or www.hrsa.gov/cicp.	• Previously vaccinated* with 1 dose of any Pfizer-BioNTech: 2-dose series of updated (2023–2024 Formula) Pfizer-BioNTech at 0, 4 weeks (minimum interval between previous Pfizer-BioNTech dose and dose 1: 3 weeks).	
	• Previously vaccinated* with 2 doses of any Pfizer-BioNTech: 1 dose of updated (2023–2024 Formula) Pfizer-BioNTech at least 4 weeks after most recent dose.	

Figure 7 Notes: Recommended Adult Immunization Schedule for Ages 19 Years and Older, United States, 2024. *Source: Centers for Disease Control and Prevention (www.cdc.gov).*

Notes Recommended Adult Immunization Schedule for Ages 19 Years or Older, United States, 2024

Haemophilus influenzae type b vaccination

Special situations
- **Anatomical or functional asplenia (including sickle cell disease):** 1 dose if previously did not receive Hib vaccine; if elective splenectomy, 1 dose preferably at least 14 days before splenectomy.
- **Hematopoietic stem cell transplant (HSCT):** 3-dose series 4 weeks apart starting 6–12 months after successful transplant, regardless of Hib vaccination history.

Hepatitis A vaccination

Routine vaccination
- **Any person who is not fully vaccinated and requests vaccination** (identification of risk factor not required): 2-dose series HepA (Havrix 6–12 months apart or Vaqta 6–18 months apart [minimum interval: 6 months]) or 3-dose series HepA-HepB (Twinrix at 0, 1, 6 months [minimum interval: dose 1 to dose 2: 4 weeks / dose 2 to dose 3: 5 months])

Special situations
- **Any person who is not fully vaccinated and who is at risk for hepatitis A virus infection:** 2-dose series HepA or 3-dose series HepA-HepB as above. Risk factors for hepatitis A virus infection include:
- **Chronic liver disease** (e.g., persons with hepatitis B, hepatitis C, cirrhosis, fatty liver disease, alcoholic liver disease, autoimmune hepatitis, alanine aminotransferase [ALT] or aspartate aminotransferase [AST] level greater than twice the upper limit of normal)
- **HIV infection**
- **Men who have sex with men**
- **Injection or noninjection drug use**
- **Persons experiencing homelessness**
- **Work with hepatitis A virus in research laboratory or with nonhuman primates with hepatitis A virus infection**
- **Travel in countries with high or intermediate endemic hepatitis A** (HepA-HepB [Twinrix] may be administered on an accelerated schedule of 3 doses at 0, 7, and 21–30 days, followed by a booster dose at 12 months)
- **Close, personal contact with international adoptee** (e.g., household or regular babysitting) in first 60 days after arrival from country with high or intermediate endemic hepatitis A (administer dose 1 as soon as adoption is planned, at least 2 weeks before adoptee's arrival)
- **Pregnancy** if at risk for infection or severe outcome from infection during pregnancy
- **Settings for exposure**, including health care settings targeting services to: injection or noninjection drug users or group homes and nonresidential day care facilities for developmentally disabled persons (individual risk factor screening not required)

Hepatitis B vaccination

Routine vaccination
- **Age 19 through 59 years:** complete a 2- or 3- or 4-dose series
- 2-dose series only applies when 2 doses of Heplisav-B* are used at least 4 weeks apart
- 3-dose series Engerix-B, PreHevbrio*, or Recombivax HB at 0, 1, 6 months [minimum intervals: dose 1 to dose 2: 4 weeks / dose 2 to dose 3: 8 weeks / dose 1 to dose 3: 16 weeks])
- 3-dose series HepA-HepB (Twinrix at 0, 1, 6 months [minimum intervals: dose 1 to dose 2: 4 weeks / dose 2 to dose 3: 5 months])
- 4-dose series HepA-HepB (Twinrix) accelerated schedule of 3 doses at 0, 7, and 21–30 days, followed by a booster dose at 12 months

*Note: Heplisav-B and PreHevbrio are not recommended in pregnancy due to lack of safety data in pregnant persons.

- **Age 60 years or older without known risk factors for hepatitis B virus infection may receive a** HepB vaccine series.
- **Age 60 years or older with known risk factors for hepatitis B virus infection should receive a** HepB vaccine series.
- **Any adult age 60 years of age or older who requests** HepB vaccination should receive a HepB vaccine series.

- **Risk factors for hepatitis B virus infection include:**
- **Chronic liver disease** e.g., persons with hepatitis C, cirrhosis, fatty liver disease, alcoholic liver disease, autoimmune hepatitis, alanine aminotransferase (ALT) or aspartate aminotransferase (AST) level greater than twice the upper limit of normal
- **HIV infection**
- **Sexual exposure risk** e.g., sex partners of hepatitis B surface antigen (HBsAg)-positive persons, sexually active persons not in mutually monogamous relationships, persons seeking evaluation or treatment for a sexually transmitted infection, men who have sex with men
- **Current or recent injection drug use**
- **Percutaneous or mucosal risk for exposure to blood** e.g., household contacts of HBsAg-positive persons, residents and staff of facilities for developmentally disabled persons, health care and public safety personnel with reasonably anticipated risk for exposure to blood or blood-contaminated body fluids; persons on maintenance dialysis (including in-center or home hemodialysis and peritoneal dialysis), persons who are prediabetes, and patients with diabetes*
- **Incarceration**
- **Travel in countries with high or intermediate endemic hepatitis B**
- *Age 60 years or older with diabetes:* Based on shared clinical decision making, 2-, 3-, or 4-dose series as above.

Figure 7 Continued

Notes Recommended Adult Immunization Schedule for Ages 19 Years or Older, United States, 2024

Special situations
- **Patients on dialysis:** complete a 3- or 4-dose series
  - 3-dose series Recombivax HB at 0, 1, 6 months (Note: Use Dialysis Formulation 1 mL = 40 mcg)
  - 4-dose series Engerix-B at 0, 1, 2, and 6 months (Note: Use 2 mL dose instead of the normal adult dose of 1 mL)

Human papillomavirus vaccination

Routine vaccination
- All persons up through age 26 years: 2- or 3-dose series depending on age at initial vaccination or condition
- Age 9–14 years at initial vaccination and received 1 dose or 2 doses less than 5 months apart: 1 additional dose
- Age 9–14 years at initial vaccination and received 2 doses at least 5 months apart: HPV vaccination series complete, no additional dose needed
- Age 15 years or older at initial vaccination: 3-dose series at 0, 1–2 months, 6 months (minimum intervals: dose 1 to dose 2: 4 weeks / dose 2 to dose 3: 12 weeks / dose 1 to dose 3: 5 months; repeat dose if administered too soon)
- No additional dose recommended when any HPV vaccine series of any valency has been completed using the recommended dosing intervals.

Shared clinical decision-making
- **Adults age 27–45 years:** Based on shared clinical decision-making, complete a 2-dose series (if initiated age 9–14 years) or 3-dose series (if initiated ≥15 years)

For additional information on shared clinical decision-making for HPV, see www.cdc.gov/vaccines/hcp/admin/downloads/isd-job-aid-scdm-hpv-shared-clinical-decision-making-hpv.pdf

Special situations
- Age ranges recommended above for routine and catch-up vaccination or shared clinical decision-making also apply in special situations
- **Immunocompromising conditions, including HIV infection:** 3-dose series, even for those who initiate vaccination at age 9 through 14 years.
- **Pregnancy:** Pregnancy testing is not needed before vaccination. HPV vaccination is not recommended until after pregnancy. No intervention needed if inadvertently vaccinated while pregnant.

Influenza vaccination

Routine vaccination
- Age 19 years or older: 1 dose any influenza vaccine appropriate for age and health status annually.
- Age 65 years or older: Any one of quadrivalent high-dose inactivated influenza vaccine (HD-IIV4), quadrivalent recombinant influenza vaccine (RIV4), or quadrivalent adjuvanted inactivated influenza vaccine (aIIV4) is preferred. If none of these three vaccines are available, then any other age-appropriate influenza vaccine should be used.
- For the 2023-2024 season, see www.cdc.gov/mmwr/volumes/72/rr/rr7202a1.htm
- For the 2024-2025 season, see the 2024–2025 ACIP influenza vaccine recommendations.

Special situations
- **Close contacts (e.g., caregivers, healthcare workers) of severely immunosuppressed persons who require a protected environment:** should not receive LAIV4. If LAIV4 is given, they should avoid contact with/caring for such immunosuppressed persons for 7 days after vaccination.
- **Note:** Persons with an egg allergy can receive any influenza vaccine (egg-based and non-egg based) appropriate for age and health status.

Measles, mumps, and rubella vaccination

Routine vaccination
- No evidence of immunity to measles, mumps, or rubella: 1 dose
- **Evidence of immunity:** Born before 1957 (except for health care personnel, see below), documentation of receipt of MMR vaccine, laboratory evidence of immunity or disease (diagnosis of disease without laboratory confirmation is not evidence of immunity)

Special situations
- **Pregnancy with no evidence of immunity to rubella:** MMR contraindicated during pregnancy; after pregnancy (before discharge from health care facility), 1 dose
- Nonpregnant persons of childbearing age with no evidence of immunity to rubella: 1 dose
- HIV infection with CD4 percentages ≥15% and CD4 count ≥200 cells/mm[3] for at least 6 months and no evidence of immunity to measles, mumps, or rubella: 2-dose series at least 4 weeks apart; MMR contraindicated for HIV infection with CD4 percentage <15% or CD4 count <200 cells/mm[3]
- **Severe immunocompromising conditions:** MMR contraindicated
- Students in postsecondary educational institutions, international travelers, and household or close, personal contacts of immunocompromised persons with no evidence of immunity to measles, mumps, or rubella: 2-dose series at least 4 weeks apart if previously did not receive any doses of MMR or 1 dose if previously received 1 dose MMR
- **In mumps outbreak settings,** for information about additional doses of MMR (including 3rd dose of MMR), see www.cdc.gov/mmwr/volumes/67/wr/mm6701a7.htm

Figure 7 Continued

Notes — Recommended Adult Immunization Schedule for Ages 19 Years or Older, United States, 2024

- **Health care personnel:**
  - Born before 1957 with no evidence of immunity to measles, mumps, or rubella: Consider 2-dose series at least 4 weeks apart for protection against measles or mumps or at least 1 dose for protection against rubella
  - Born in 1957 or later with no evidence of immunity to measles, mumps, or rubella: 2-dose series at least 4 weeks apart for protection against measles or mumps or at least 1 dose for protection against rubella

Meningococcal vaccination

Special situations for MenACWY
- Anatomical or functional asplenia (including sickle cell disease), HIV infection, persistent complement component deficiency, complement inhibitor (e.g., eculizumab, ravulizumab) use: 2-dose series at least 8 weeks apart and revaccinate every 5 years if risk remains
- Travel in countries with hyperendemic or epidemic meningococcal disease, or microbiologists routinely exposed to *Neisseria meningitidis*: 1 dose MenACWY (Menveo or MenQuadfi) and revaccinate every 5 years if risk remains
- First-year college students who live in residential housing (if not previously vaccinated at age 16 years or older) or military recruits: 1 dose MenACWY (Menveo or MenQuadfi)
- For MenACWY booster dose recommendations for groups listed under "Special situations" and in an outbreak setting (e.g., in community or organizational settings, or among men who have sex with men) and additional meningococcal vaccination information, see www.cdc.gov/mmwr/volumes/69/rr/rr6909a1.htm

Shared clinical decision-making for MenB
- Adolescents and young adults age 16–23 years (age 16–18 years preferred) not at increased risk for meningococcal disease: Based on shared clinical decision-making, 2-dose series MenB-4C (Bexsero) at least 1 month apart or 2-dose series MenB-FHbp (Trumenba) at 0, 6 months (if dose 2 was administered less than 6 months after dose 1, administer dose 3 at least 4 months after dose 2); MenB-4C and MenB-FHbp are not interchangeable (use same product for all doses in series).

For additional information on shared clinical decision-making for MenB, see www.cdc.gov/vaccines/hcp/admin/downloads/isd-job-aid-scdm-mening-b-shared-clinical-decision-making.pdf

Special situations for MenB
- Anatomical or functional asplenia (including sickle cell disease), persistent complement component deficiency, complement inhibitor (e.g., eculizumab, ravulizumab) use, or microbiologists routinely exposed to *Neisseria meningitidis*:
2-dose primary series MenB-4C (Bexsero) at least 1 month apart or 3-dose primary series MenB-FHbp (Trumenba) at 0, 1–2, 6 months (if dose 2 was administered at least 6 months after dose 1, dose 3 not needed; if dose 3 is administered earlier than 4 months after dose 2, a fourth dose should be administered at least 4 months after dose 3); MenB-4C and MenB-FHbp are not interchangeable (use same product for all doses in series); 1 dose MenB booster 1 year after primary series and revaccinate every 2–3 years if risk remains.
- Pregnancy: Delay MenB until after pregnancy unless at increased risk and vaccination benefits outweigh potential risks.
- For MenB booster dose recommendations for groups listed under "Special situations" and in an outbreak setting (e.g., in community or organizational settings and among men who have sex with men) and additional meningococcal vaccination information, see www.cdc.gov/mmwr/volumes/69/rr/rr6909a1.htm

Note: MenB vaccines may be administered simultaneously with MenACWY vaccines if indicated, but at a different anatomic site, if feasible.

Adults may receive a single dose of Penbraya as an alternative to separate administration of MenACWY and MenB when both vaccines would be given on the same clinic day. For adults not at increased risk, if Penbraya is used for dose 1 MenB, MenB-FHbp (Trumenba) should be administered for dose 2 MenB. For adults at increased risk of meningococcal disease, Penbraya may be used for additional MenACWY and MenB doses (including booster doses) if both would be given on the same clinic day **and** at least 6 months have elapsed since most recent Penbraya dose.

Mpox vaccination

Special situations
- Any person at risk for Mpox infection: 2-dose series, 28 days apart.

Risk factors for Mpox infection include:
- Persons who are gay, bisexual, and other MSM, transgender or nonbinary people who in the past 6 months have had:
  A new diagnosis of at least 1 sexually transmitted disease
  More than 1 sex partner
  Sex at a commercial sex venue
  Sex in association with a large public event in a geographic area where Mpox transmission is occurring
- Persons who are sexual partners of the persons described above
- Persons who anticipate experiencing any of the situations described above

Figure 7 Continued

Notes Recommended Adult Immunization Schedule for Ages 19 Years or Older, United States, 2024

- **Pregnancy:** There is currently no ACIP recommendation for Jynneos use in pregnancy due to lack of safety data in pregnant persons. Pregnant persons with any risk factor described above may receive Jynneos.
- **Healthcare personnel:** Except in rare circumstances (e.g. no available personal protective equipment), healthcare personnel who do not have any of the sexual risk factors described above should not receive Jynneos.

For detailed information, see: www.cdc.gov/vaccines/acip/meetings/downloads/slides-2023-10-25-26/04-MPOX-Rao-508.pdf

Pneumococcal vaccination

Routine vaccination
- **Age 65 years or older who have:**
- **Not previously received a dose of PCV13, PCV15, or PCV20 or whose previous vaccination history is unknown:** 1 dose PCV15 OR 1 dose PCV20.
 - If PCV15 is used, administer 1 dose PPSV23 at least 1 year after the PCV15 dose (may use minimum interval of 8 weeks for adults with an immunocompromising condition,* cochlear implant, or cerebrospinal fluid leak).
- **Previously received only PCV13:** follow the recommendation above.
- **Previously received only PCV15:** 1 dose PCV20 OR 1 dose PPSV23.
 - If PCV20 is selected, administer at least 1 year after the last PCV13 dose.
 - If PPSV23 is selected, administer at least 1 year after the last PCV13 dose (may use minimum interval of 8 weeks for adults with an immunocompromising condition,* cochlear implant, or cerebrospinal fluid leak).
- **Previously received only PPSV23:** 1 dose PCV15 OR 1 dose PCV20. Administer either PCV15 or PCV20 at least 1 year after the last PPSV23 dose.
 - If PCV15 is used, no additional PPSV23 doses are recommended.
- **Previously received both PCV13 and PPSV23 but NO PPSV23 was received at age 65 years or older:** 1 dose PCV20 OR 1 dose PPSV23.
 - If PCV20 is selected, administer at least 5 years after the last pneumococcal vaccine dose.
 - If PPSV23 is selected, see dosing schedule at www.cdc.gov/vaccines/vpd/pneumo/downloads/pneumo-vaccine-timing.pdf.
- **Previously received both PCV13 and PPSV23, AND PPSV23 was received at age 65 years or older:** Based on shared clinical decision-making, 1 dose of PCV20 at least 5 years after the last pneumococcal vaccine dose.
- For guidance on determining which pneumococcal vaccines a patient needs and when, please refer to the mobile app, which can be downloaded here: www.cdc.gov/vaccines/vpd/pneumo/hcp/pneumoapp.html.

Special situations
- **Age 19–64 years with certain underlying medical conditions or other risk factors** who have:**
- **Not previously received a PCV13, PCV15, or PCV20 or whose previous vaccination history is unknown:** 1 dose PCV15 OR 1 dose PCV20.
 - If PCV15 is used, administer 1 dose PPSV23 at least 1 year after the PCV15 dose (may use minimum interval of 8 weeks for adults with an immunocompromising condition,* cochlear implant, or cerebrospinal fluid leak).
- **Previously received only PCV7:** follow the recommendation above.
- **Previously received only PCV13:** 1 dose PCV20 OR 1 dose PPSV23.
 - If PCV20 is selected, administer at least 1 year after the PCV13 dose.
 - If PPSV23 is selected, see dosing schedule at www.cdc.gov/vaccines/vpd/pneumo/downloads/pneumo-vaccine-timing.pdf
- **Previously received only PPSV23:** 1 dose PCV15 OR 1 dose PCV20. Administer either PCV15 or PCV20 at least 1 year after the last PPSV23 dose.
 - If PCV15 is used, no additional PPSV23 doses are recommended.
- **Previously received PCV13 and 1 dose of PPSV23:** 1 dose PCV20 OR 1 dose PPSV23.
 - If PCV20 is selected, administer at least 5 years after the last pneumococcal vaccine dose.
 - If PPSV23 is selected, see dosing schedule at www.cdc.gov/vaccines/vpd/pneumo/downloads/pneumo-vaccine-timing.pdf
- For guidance on determining which pneumococcal vaccines a patient needs and when, please refer to the mobile app which can be downloaded here: www.cdc.gov/vaccines/vpd/pneumo/hcp/pneumoapp.html

*Note: Immunocompromising conditions include chronic renal failure, nephrotic syndrome, immunodeficiencies, iatrogenic immunosuppression, generalized malignancy, HIV infection, Hodgkin disease, leukemia, lymphoma, multiple myeloma, solid organ transplant, congenital or acquired asplenia, or sickle cell disease or other hemoglobinopathies.

**Note: Underlying medical conditions or other risk factors include alcoholism, chronic heart/liver/lung disease, chronic renal failure, cigarette smoking, CSF leak, diabetes mellitus, generalized malignancy, HIV infection, Hodgkin disease, immunodeficiencies, iatrogenic immunosuppression, leukemia, lymphoma, multiple myeloma, nephrotic syndrome, solid organ transplant, or sickle cell disease or other hemoglobinopathies.

Poliovirus vaccination

Routine vaccination
- **Adults known or suspected to be unvaccinated or incompletely vaccinated:** administer remaining doses (1, 2, or 3 IPV doses) to complete a 3-dose primary series.* Unless there are specific reasons to believe they were not vaccinated, most adults who were born and raised in the United States can assume they were vaccinated against polio as children.

Figure 7 Continued

Notes Recommended Adult Immunization Schedule for Ages 19 Years or Older, United States, 2024

Special situations
- **Adults at increased risk of exposure to poliovirus who completed primary series***: may administer one lifetime IPV booster

  *Note: Complete primary series consists of at least 3 doses of IPV or trivalent oral poliovirus vaccine (tOPV) in any combination.

  For detailed information, see: www.cdc.gov/vaccines/vpd/polio/hcp/recommendations.html

Respiratory syncytial virus vaccination

Routine vaccination
- **Pregnant at 32 weeks 0 days through 36 weeks and 6 days gestation from September through January in most of the continental United States***: 1 dose RSV vaccine (Abrysvo™). Administer RSV vaccine regardless of previous RSV infection.
  - Either maternal RSV vaccination or infant immunization with nirsevimab (RSV monoclonal antibody) is recommended to prevent respiratory syncytial virus lower respiratory tract infection in infants.
- **All other pregnant persons**: RSV vaccine not recommended

  There is currently no ACIP recommendation for RSV vaccination in subsequent pregnancies. No data are available to inform whether additional doses are needed in later pregnancies.

Special situations
- **Age 60 years or older**: Based on shared clinical decision-making, 1 dose RSV vaccine (Arexvy® or Abrysvo™). Persons most likely to benefit from vaccination are those considered to be at increased risk for severe RSV disease.** For additional information on shared clinical decision-making for RSV in older adults, see www.cdc.gov/vaccines/vpd/rsv/downloads/provider-job-aid-for-older-adults-508.pdf

  For further guidance, see www.cdc.gov/mmwr/volumes/72/wr/mm7229a4.htm

  *Note: Providers in jurisdictions with RSV seasonality that differs from most of the continental United States (e.g., Alaska, jurisdiction with tropical climate) should follow guidance from public health authorities (e.g., CDC, health departments) or regional medical centers on timing of administration based on local RSV seasonality. Refer to the 2024 Child and Adolescent Immunization Schedule for considerations regarding nirsevimab administration to infants.

  **Note: Adults age 60 years or older who are at increased risk for severe RSV disease include those with chronic medical conditions such as lung diseases (e.g., chronic obstructive pulmonary disease, asthma), cardiovascular diseases (e.g., congestive heart failure, coronary artery disease), neurologic or neuromuscular conditions, kidney disorders, liver disorders, hematologic disorders, diabetes mellitus, and moderate or severe immune compromise (either attributable to a medical condition or receipt of immunosuppressive medications or treatment); those who are considered to be frail; those of advanced age; those who reside in nursing homes or other long-term care facilities; and those with other underlying medical conditions or factors that a health care provider determines might increase the risk of severe respiratory disease.

Tetanus, diphtheria, and pertussis vaccination

Routine vaccination
- **Previously did not receive Tdap at or after age 11 years***: 1 dose Tdap, then Td or Tdap every 10 years
- **Previously did not receive primary vaccination series for tetanus, diphtheria, or pertussis**: 1 dose Tdap followed by 1 dose Td or Tdap at least 4 weeks later, and a third dose of Td or Tdap 6–12 months later (Tdap is preferred as first dose and can be substituted for any Td dose), Td or Tdap every 10 years thereafter.
- **Pregnancy**: 1 dose Tdap during each pregnancy, preferably in early part of gestational weeks 27–36.

- **Wound management**: Persons with 3 or more doses of tetanus-toxoid-containing vaccine: For clean and minor wounds, administer Tdap or Td if more than 10 years since last dose of tetanus-toxoid-containing vaccine; for all other wounds, administer Tdap or Td if more than 5 years since last dose of tetanus-toxoid-containing vaccine. Tdap is preferred for persons who have not previously received Tdap or whose Tdap history is unknown. If a tetanus-toxoid-containing vaccine is indicated for a pregnant woman, use Tdap. For detailed information, see www.cdc.gov/mmwr/volumes/69/wr/mm6903a5.htm

  *Note: Tdap administered at age 10 years may be counted as the adolescent dose recommended at age 11-12 years

Varicella vaccination

Routine vaccination
- **No evidence of immunity to varicella**: 2-dose series 4–8 weeks apart; if previously did not receive varicella-containing vaccine (VAR or MMRV [measles-mumps-rubella-varicella vaccine] for children); if previously received 1 dose varicella-containing vaccine, 1 dose at least 4 weeks after first dose.
- **Evidence of immunity**: U.S.-born before 1980 (except for pregnant persons and health care personnel [see below]), documentation of 2 doses varicella-containing vaccine at least 4 weeks apart, diagnosis or verification of history of varicella or herpes zoster by a health care provider, laboratory evidence of immunity or disease.

Special situations
- **Pregnancy with no evidence of immunity to varicella**: VAR contraindicated during pregnancy; after pregnancy (before discharge from health care facility), 1 dose if previously received 1 dose varicella-containing vaccine or dose 1 of 2-dose series (dose 2, 4–8 weeks later) if previously did not receive any varicella-containing vaccine, regardless of whether U.S.-born before 1980.

Figure 7 Continued

Notes Recommended Adult Immunization Schedule for Ages 19 Years or Older, United States, 2024

- **Health care personnel with no evidence of immunity to varicella:** 1 dose if previously received 1 dose varicella-containing vaccine; 2-dose series 4–8 weeks apart if previously did not receive any varicella-containing vaccine, regardless of whether U.S.-born before 1980.
- **HIV infection with CD4 percentages ≥15% and CD4 count ≥200 cells/mm³ with no evidence of immunity:** Vaccination may be considered (2 doses 3 months apart); VAR contraindicated for HIV infection with CD4 percentage <15% or CD4 count <200 cells/mm³
- **Severe immunocompromising conditions:** VAR contraindicated.
- **Immunocompromising conditions (including persons with HIV regardless of CD4 count)**:** 2-dose series recombinant zoster vaccine (RZV, Shingrix) 2–6 months apart (minimum interval: 4 weeks; repeat dose if administered too soon). For detailed information, see www.cdc.gov/shingles/vaccination/immunocompromised-adults.html

****Note:** If there is no documented history of varicella, varicella vaccination, or herpes zoster, providers should refer to the clinical considerations for use of RZV in immunocompromised adults aged ≥19 years and the ACIP varicella vaccine recommendations for further guidance: www.cdc.gov/mmwr/volumes/71/wr/mm7103a2.htm

Zoster vaccination

Routine vaccination

- **Age 50 years or older*:** 2-dose series recombinant zoster vaccine (RZV, Shingrix) 2–6 months apart (minimum interval: 4 weeks; repeat dose if administered too soon), regardless of previous herpes zoster or history of zoster vaccine live (ZVL, Zostavax) vaccination.

***Note:** Serologic evidence of prior varicella is not necessary for zoster vaccination. However, if serologic evidence of varicella susceptibility becomes available, providers should follow ACIP guidelines for varicella vaccination first. RZV is not indicated for the prevention of varicella, and there are limited data on the use of RZV in persons without a history of varicella or varicella vaccination.

Special situations

- **Pregnancy:** There is currently no ACIP recommendation for RZV use in pregnancy. Consider delaying RZV until after pregnancy.

Figure 7 Continued

SUMMARY OF VACCINES ROUTINELY RECOMMENDED FOR INFANTS, CHILDREN, AND ADULTS

Table 6 summarizes the vaccines that are routinely recommended for infants, children, and adults.

Table 6 SUMMARY OF VACCINES ROUTINELY RECOMMENDED FOR INFANTS, CHILDREN, AND ADULTS

Vaccine	Age Group	Dosing
Td/Tdap (tetanus, diphtheria, acellular pertussis)	19 years of age and older	1 dose of Tdap; Tdap booster every 8–10 years; pregnant women should receive a Tdap dose with each pregnancy
DTaP	6 weeks to <7 years of age	5 doses (2, 4, 6, 15–18 months of age, 4–6 years of age)
IPV	6 weeks of age and older	4 doses (2, 4, 6–18 months of age, 4–6 years of age)
Rotavirus	2 months and older	2 doses (2, 4 months of age) if RV1 3 doses (2, 4, 6 months of age) if RV5
Haemophilus influenzae type b	6 weeks and older	2- or 3-dose primary series (2, 4, 6 months of age) depending on vaccine 12 to 15 month of age booster dose

Influenza	All persons ≥6 months of age	1 dose annually
MMR (measles, mumps, rubella)	If born in 1957 or later (for those with no documentation of vaccination or clinical disease)	1–2 doses (0, 4–8 weeks)
	12 months and older	2 doses (12–15 months of age, 4–6 years of age)
Varicella	All persons ≥7 year of age lacking documentation of vaccination or clinical disease	2 doses (0, 4–8 weeks after first dose)
	12 months and older	2 doses (12–15 months of age, 4–6 years of age)
Herpes zoster (shingles)	Persons ≥50 years of age with or without history of herpes zoster or prior vaccination	2 doses (0, 2–6 months after first dose)
	Persons ≥19 years of age who are or will be immunodeficient or immunosuppressed because of disease or therapy	
Pneumococcal polysaccharide (PPSV23)	Persons 2 years of age to 64 years in at-risk groups	1–2 doses (separated by 5 years)
	Persons ≥65 years	1 dose

(continued)

Table 6 CONTINUED

Vaccine	Age Group	Dosing
Pneumococcal conjugate (PCV15* and PCV20)	Persons ≥19 years of age with at-risk conditions	1 dose
	Persons ≥65 years	1 dose
		*If persons have not received PPSV23 in past and PCV15 is given, a dose of PPSV23 is given ≥8 weeks after the dose of PCV15.
	6 weeks of age and older	3-dose primary series (2, 4, 6 months of age), booster dose (12–15 months of age)
Hepatitis A	All children ≥1 year, all persons in at-risk groups or travelers	2 doses (0, 6–18 months after first dose)
Hepatitis B	All infants and children beginning at birth, persons in at-risk groups, travelers of any age	3 doses (0, 1, 6 months) OR
	All adults 19 to 59 years of age	2 doses (0, 1 month after first dose) HepB-CpG (18 years of age and older) OR
		3 doses (0, 1, 6 months) or (0, 7, 21–30 days and booster at 12 months) HepA/HepB

HPV	All persons 9 to 14 years of age	2 doses (0 and 6–12 months)
	Persons 15 to 26 years of age and immunocompromised	3 doses (0, 1–2, and 6 months)
	Some adults age 27 through 45 years (shared clinical decision-making)	
Meningococcal quadrivalent conjugate (MenACWY)	Adolescents	1–3 doses
	Persons in at-risk groups and travelers 9 months of age and older	1 or more doses
Meningococcal pentavalent conjugate (PENBRAYA)	Persons 10 through 25 years of age.	2 doses (0, 6 months)
Meningococcal B (MenB)	16 to 24 years	MenB-4C (2 doses separated by at least 1 month)
		MenB FHbp (2 doses separated by 6 months)

(continued)

Table 6 CONTINUED

Vaccine	Age Group	Dosing
Mpox	Adults 18 years of age and older determined to be at high risk for monkeypox infection	2 doses (0, 1 month)
RSV	≥60 years of age (adjuvanted and non-adjuvanted vaccines)	1 dose
	Pregnant women (non-adjuvanted vaccine)	1 dose
COVID-19	6 months to <5 years of age NOT immunocompromised	Unvaccinated 1. Two-dose primary series of 2023–2024 Moderna vaccine with 4 to 8 weeks between dose 1 and dose 2 2. Three-dose primary series of Pfizer–BioNTech 2023–2024 vaccine with 3 to 8 weeks between dose 1 and dose 2 and at least 8 weeks between dose 2 and dose 3 Vaccinated 1. Received 1 dose of any Moderna vaccine in past: Give 1 dose 2023–2024 Moderna vaccine if 4 to 8 weeks after last vaccine dose.

2. Received 2 or more doses of any Moderna vaccine in past: Give 1 dose 2023–2024 Moderna vaccine if at least 8 weeks after last vaccine dose.

3. Received 1 dose of any Pfizer–BioNTech vaccine in past: Give 2 doses 2023–2024 Pfizer–BioNTech vaccine if 3 to 8 weeks after last vaccine dose. There should be at least an 8-week interval between dose 1 and dose 2.

4. Received 2 or more doses of any Pfizer–BioNTech vaccine in past: Give 1 dose of 2023–2024 Pfizer–BioNTech vaccine if at least 8 weeks since last vaccine dose.

≥5 years of age NOT immunocompromised

Single dose of 2023–2024 Moderna or Pfizer–BioNTech COVID-19 vaccine (both unvaccinated and previously vaccinated)

≥12 years of age NOT immunocompromised

May also use Novavax COVID-19 vaccine

(continued)

Table 6 CONTINUED

Vaccine	Age Group	Dosing
		Unvaccinated
		2 doses of 2023–2024 Novavax vaccine with 3 to 8 weeks between dose 1 and dose 2
		Vaccinated
		1 dose of 2023–2024 Novavax vaccine if at least 8 weeks since last vaccine dose of any COVID-19 vaccine
	6 months to 4 years of age with moderate to severe immunocompromise	Unvaccinated
		1. Three-dose primary series 2023–2024 Moderna vaccine with 4 weeks between dose 1 and dose 2 and at least 4 weeks between dose 2 and does 3
		2. Three-dose primary series 2023–2024 Pfizer–BioNTech vaccine with 3 weeks between dose 1 and dose 2 and at least 8 weeks between dose 2 and dose 3

Vaccinated

1. Received 1 dose of any Moderna vaccine in past: Give 2 doses of 2023–2024 Moderna vaccine if at least 4 weeks after last vaccine dose and at least 4 weeks between dose 1 and dose 2.

2. Received 2 doses of any Moderna vaccine in past: Give 1 dose of 2023–2024 Moderna vaccine if at least 4 weeks after last dose.

3. Received 3 or more doses of any Moderna vaccine in past: Give 1 dose of 2023–2024 Moderna vaccine if at least 8 weeks after last dose.

4. Received 1 dose of any Pfizer–BioNTech vaccine in past. Give 2 doses of 2023–2024 Pfizer–BioNTech vaccine if at least 3 weeks after last vaccine dose and at least 8 weeks between dose 1 and dose 2.

5. Received 2 or more doses of any Pfizer–BioNTech vaccine in past: Give 1 dose of 2023–2024 Pfizer–BioNTech vaccine if at least 8 weeks after last vaccine dose.

(continued)

Table 6 CONTINUED

Vaccine	Age Group	Dosing
	5 to 11 years of age with moderate to severe immunocompromise	Unvaccinated 1. Three doses of Moderna 2023–2024 vaccine with 4 weeks between dose 1 and dose 2 and at least 4 weeks between dose 2 and dose 3 2. Three doses of Pfizer–BioNTech 2023–2024 vaccine with 3 weeks between dose 1 and dose 2 and at least 4 weeks between dose 2 and dose 3 Previously vaccinated 1. Received 1 dose of any Moderna vaccine in past: Give 2 doses of 2023–2024 Moderna vaccine if 4 weeks after last vaccine dose and at least 4 weeks between dose 1 and dose 2. 2. Received 2 doses of any Moderna vaccine in past: Give 1 dose of 2023–2024 Moderna vaccine if at least 4 weeks after last vaccine dose.

3. Received 1 dose of any Pfizer–BioNTech vaccine in past: Give 2 doses of 2023–2024 Pfizer–BioNTech vaccine if at least 3 weeks after last dose and at least 4 weeks between dose 1 and dose 2.

4. Received 2 doses of any Pfizer–BioNTech vaccine in past: Give 1 dose of 2023–2024 Pfizer–BioNTech vaccine if at least 4 weeks after last vaccine dose.

5. Received ≥3 doses of any mRNA vaccine in past: Give 1 dose of 2023–2024 Moderna or 1 dose of 2023–2024 Pfizer–BioNTech vaccine if at least 8 weeks after last vaccine dose.

Unvaccinated

1. Three doses of 2023–2024 Moderna vaccine with 4 weeks between dose 1 and dose 2 and at least 4 weeks between dose 2 and dose 3

2. Three doses of 2023–2024 Pfizer–BioNTech vaccine with 3 weeks between dose 1 and dose 2 and at least 4 weeks between dose 2 and dose 3

≥12 years with moderate to severe immunocompromise

(continued)

55

Table 6 CONTINUED

Vaccine	Age Group	Dosing
		3. Two doses of Novovax vaccine with 3 weeks between dose 1 and dose 2
	Previously vaccinated	1. Received 1 dose of any Moderna vaccine in past: Give 2 doses of 2023–2024 Moderna vaccine if at least 4 weeks after last vaccine dose and at least 4 weeks between dose 1 and dose 2.
		2. Received 2 doses of any Moderna vaccine in past: Give 1 dose of 2023–2024 Moderna vaccine if at least 4 weeks after last vaccine dose.
		3. Received 1 dose of any Pfizer–BioNTech vaccine in past: Give 2 doses of 2023-2024 Pfizer–BioNTech vaccine if 3 weeks after last vaccine dose with at least 4 weeks between dose 1 and dose 2.
		4. Received 2 doses of any Pfizer–BioNTech vaccine in past: Give 1 dose of 2023–2024 Pfizer–BioNTech vaccine if at least 4 weeks after last vaccine dose.

5. Received ≥3 doses of any mRNA vaccine in past: Give 1 dose of 2023–2024 Moderna or 1 dose of 2023–2024 Pfizer–BioNTech vaccine if at least 8 weeks after last vaccine dose.

6. Received 1 or more doses of Novavax or Janssen, including in combination with any mRNA vaccine dose(s): Give 1 dose of 2023–2024 Moderna or 1 dose of 2023–2024 Pfizer–BioNTech vaccine if at least 8 weeks after last vaccine dose.

VACCINES AND PREGNANCY

Did you know that:

- During the 1917–1918 influenza pandemic in Chicago, the mortality rate was 45% among hospitalized pregnant women with influenza.
- During the 2009 H1N1 influenza pandemic, pregnant women made up 1% of the U.S. population but accounted for 5% of the deaths from the H1N1 influenza virus. More than 91% of the deaths occurred during the second and third trimesters of pregnancy.
- If a woman contracts rubella during the first 10 weeks of pregnancy, the rate of transmission to the developing fetus is as high as 90%.
- The damage caused by a congenital rubella infection does not stop at birth; glaucoma, cataracts, retinal detachment, esophageal problems, autism, and thyroiditis may occur later in life.
- COVID-19 infection, caused by the SARS–CoV-2 virus, during pregnancy increases the risk of delivering a preterm (earlier than 37 weeks) or stillborn infant. Women who are pregnant or recently pregnant are more likely to get very sick from COVID-19 compared to people who are not pregnant. People with COVID-19 during pregnancy may also be more likely to have other pregnancy complications.

Many infectious diseases are particularly threatening when they occur during pregnancy because of the serious complication rates that approach levels associated with those of high-risk populations. Many of these diseases are vaccine-preventable ones, some of which can directly affect a fetus at various stages of pregnancy.

The use of vaccines during pregnancy poses only theoretical risks to the developing fetus. There is no evidence indicating that vaccines currently in use have detrimental effects on the fetus; however, the traditional approach to using vaccines during pregnancy has been that pregnant women should receive a vaccine only when the vaccine is unlikely to cause harm, risk of disease exposure is high, and the infection would pose a significant risk to the pregnant woman, fetus, or newborn infant. Four vaccines are now recommended for routine administration during pregnancy in the United States: inactivated influenza vaccines, Tdap vaccine, COVID-19 vaccine, and RSV vaccine. Diphtheria and tetanus toxoids (Td vaccine) and pneumococcal vaccine (polysaccharide or conjugate) may be indicated in some circumstances.

The American Congress of Obstetricians and Gynecologists (ACOG) and the Advisory Committee for Immunization Practice of the Centers for Disease Control and Prevention (CDC) have made strong recommendations for the use of vaccinations to improve the health of both mothers and infants. Table 7 details the vaccines that are routinely recommended, contraindicated, not recommended, or may be given in certain circumstances during pregnancy. Details of the individual vaccine-preventable diseases are given in the specific vaccine sections of this book.

Specific Complications of Vaccine-Preventable Diseases in Pregnant Women and Preventative Vaccines and Their Use

Tdap (Tetanus, Diphtheria, Acellular Pertussis)
A tetanus-containing vaccine can be given if indicated at any time during pregnancy, and the current recommendation is that it should be given as Tdap vaccine, as noted below.

Table 7 VACCINES DURING PREGNANCY

Vaccines Routinely Given to Pregnant Women	Vaccines Contraindicated During Pregnancy	Vaccines Not Recommended During Pregnancy	Vaccines Given in Certain Circumstances During Pregnancy
Td (late second or third trimester)	MMR	HPV	Hepatitis A
Tdap (late second or third trimester)	Live, attenuated, intranasal influenza (LAIV)	Mpox	Hepatitis B
Inactivated injectable influenza (any trimester of pregnancy)	Varicella		Pneumococcal polysaccharide or pneumococcal conjugate
	Dengue		Meningococcal quadrivalent conjugate
COVID-19 mRNA vaccines (any trimester of pregnancy)			Meningococcal B
			IPV
RSV (between 32 and 36 weeks of gestation)			Cholera

Pertussis (whooping cough) is particularly severe in infants especially during the first 3 months of life, when the vast majority of deaths from the disease occur. These infants are either too young to be immunized or have only received 1 dose of a pertussis-containing vaccine and have little or no immunity against the disease. The disease is transmitted from any close contact, particularly family members (especially mothers, fathers, grandparents, and older siblings), caregivers (nannies, babysitters, day care providers), and visitors (aunts, uncles, friends). Infants begin their primary immunization schedule at 2 months of age when they receive their first dose of pertussis-containing vaccine. The primary immunization schedule consists of 3 doses of a pertussis-containing vaccine that is given at 2, 4, and 6 months of age. This leaves infants younger than age 3 months at high risk for serious complications of the disease. To provide maximum protection to this young infant population, it is recommended that a pregnant woman receive a dose of Tdap vaccine during the late second or third trimester (between 27 and 36 weeks) of *each* pregnancy. If she was not immunized during the pregnancy and she has never received a prior dose of Tdap vaccine, she should receive the vaccine postpartum, as a one-time, single dose, as soon as possible after delivery and before leaving the hospital. She should be revaccinated with a dose of Tdap in all subsequent pregnancies.

It is also extremely important to vaccinate all susceptible family members and household contacts as well as other persons who have regular contact with the young infants, including day care providers, nannies, family members, and visitors, in order to prevent them from contracting pertussis. This protection cocoons the infant who is too young to be immunized and prevents the spread of the disease. Health care workers who will have any direct contact with a patient should also be immunized.

Influenza
Pregnant women often have the highest rates of serious disease, complications, hospitalizations, and deaths from influenza.

Pregnancy itself is considered an indication for influenza vaccination. The risk of hospitalization for heart and lung problems is more than four times higher in pregnant women compared to nonpregnant women, and the risk increases exponentially as pregnancy progresses. The rate of complications in otherwise healthy pregnant women is similar to that of the high-risk nonpregnant patient. This risk is further increased in women with asthma who are pregnant. During the 2009 H1N1 epidemic, infected pregnant women were at very high risk for severe or fatal illness and were at significantly increased risk for fetal death, spontaneous abortion, and preterm delivery. Secondary bacterial pneumonia occurred much more commonly in this population and may be necrotizing, most often due to *Staphylococcus aureus* and *Streptococcus pneumoniae*. It is safe for a woman to receive all routine vaccines (both inactivated and live) immediately after giving birth; breastfeeding is not a precaution or contraindication to receiving a vaccine.

Several different formulations and methods of administration for influenza vaccine are available and are discussed in this book. All influenza vaccines contain the same four influenza strains that change on an annual basis. Only the inactivated injectable influenza vaccines are recommended to be given during pregnancy. ACOG strongly recommends that *all* women who will be pregnant during influenza season receive a dose of influenza vaccine. The vaccine may be given during *any* trimester of pregnancy.

COVID-19

Women who are pregnant or were recently pregnant are more likely to get severely ill from COVID-19 compared to people who are not pregnant. Pregnancy causes changes in the body that could make it easier to get very sick from respiratory viruses such as the one that causes COVID-19, and these changes in the body can continue after pregnancy. Women in the late second or third trimester who become ill with COVID-19 are at increased risk for developing severe illness that may require hospitalization, admission to an intensive care unit, or a ventilator or other special equipment to help them breathe, and they are also at increased risk of death.

Other factors can further increase the risk for getting very sick from COVID-19 during or recently after pregnancy include having certain underlying medical conditions (cancer, chronic kidney and liver disease, chronic lung disease including asthma, diabetes types 1 and 2, heart conditions, HIV, conditions causing a weakened immune system, being overweight or obese, age 35 years or older, sickle cell disease and thalassemia, current or former cigarette smoker, and having a substance use disorder), living or working in a community with high numbers of COVID-19 cases and low levels of COVID-19 vaccination, and belonging to some racial and ethnic minority groups that may be at increased risk of getting sick from COVID-19 because of health inequities that they face.

People with COVID-19 during pregnancy are more likely to experience complications that can affect their pregnancy and developing infant compared to people without COVID-19 during pregnancy. COVID-19 during pregnancy increases the risk of delivering a preterm (earlier than 37 weeks) or stillborn infant and is more likely to cause other pregnancy complications.

COVID-19 vaccination is recommended for all people who are pregnant, breastfeeding, or trying to get pregnant now or might become pregnant in the future. mRNA COVID-19 vaccines are preferred over other COVID-19 vaccines and may be administered during any trimester of pregnancy. There is no evidence of adverse maternal or fetal effects from vaccinating pregnant individuals with the COVID-19 vaccine.

Respiratory Syncytial Virus
Respiratory syncytial virus (RSV) is the most common cause of acute lower respiratory tract illness and a leading cause of death in infants younger than age 6 months. Severe RSV disease peaks in the first 2 or 3 months of life. Maternal vaccination with RSV vaccine provides transplacental transfer of maternal antibodies to the fetus, providing protection to the infant immediately after birth and during the first months of life.

RSVpreF vaccine is recommended to be given to pregnant women between 32 and 36 weeks of gestation at the beginning of and during RSV season. The vaccine has been shown to be safe and effective. This recommendation is supported by ACOG, the CDC, and the American Academy of Pediatrics.

Measles, Mumps, and Rubella

Rubeola (Measles)
This is usually a mild disease in children; however, in adults it can be associated with serious complications, including pneumonia, encephalitis, and death. In pregnancy, it can cause abortion, prematurity, and low birth weight. Immunity is important because the disease is highly contagious; easily spread from an infected person; and can be imported from other countries where vaccination is not routinely recommended, as in the United States. Unvaccinated travelers returning from countries where vaccination is not widely done present significant risk to their community, particularly where there has been opposition to appropriate vaccination program.

Mumps
Mumps manifests as salivary gland swelling and tenderness; it has long been associated with orchitis and potential male infertility.

However, oophoritis can occur in females, also potentially reducing fertility. Early in pregnancy, there is the possibility of spontaneous abortion. When the disease occurs late in pregnancy, there is the potential for preterm birth and low-birth-weight infants.

Rubella

Rubella was the first virus demonstrated as a teratogen, and there is a high risk of developing congenital rubella syndrome (CRS) if the infection occurs in the first trimester of pregnancy. The classic triad of CRS includes deafness, cataracts, and cardiac disease. Rubella infection in the mother may be asymptomatic or mildly symptomatic but can cross the placental barrier and cause defects in the developing fetus.

MMR (Measles, Mumps, Rubella) Vaccine

This is a live, attenuated virus vaccine; administration is contraindicated during pregnancy. Susceptibility can be tested prior to the onset of pregnancy, particularly if the woman does not have proof of having had rubella disease or immunization. All women of childbearing age should be immunized. The patient should wait 1 month after vaccination to become pregnant. If the vaccine is given inadvertently in pregnancy, termination should *not* be recommended because there is no evidence of effect on the fetus or clinical rubella in infants born to pregnant women who were inadvertently vaccinated. Postpartum, susceptible women should be immunized; there is no contraindication to vaccination with breastfeeding.

Varicella

Because the effects of the varicella virus on the fetus are unknown, pregnant women should not be vaccinated. Nonpregnant women who are vaccinated should avoid becoming pregnant for 1 month after each vaccine dose. For persons without evidence of immunity, having a pregnant household member is not a contraindication for vaccination.

Hepatitis A

Hepatitis A causes fever, nausea, abdominal pain, and jaundice as a result of an acute, self-limiting liver infection. The virus is transmitted via the fecal–oral route after close contact with infected individuals or contaminated food or drinks. Although there are insufficient data to conclude that the vaccine is safe during pregnancy, there is no live virus component in the vaccine, so it is unlikely to cause harm to either the mother or fetus, and pregnant women should receive the vaccine if they are at high risk for infection.

Hepatitis B

Hepatitis B virus causes acute liver infection with inflammation, vomiting, and jaundice. It can be self-limited or result in chronic hepatitis associated with long-term sequelae, including cirrhosis, liver failure, hepatocellular carcinoma, and death. The virus is transmitted by close contact with infected blood and body fluids.

Hepatitis B infection in pregnancy, both acute and chronic infection, is concerning because of the risk of vertical transmission to the fetus and newborn. All pregnant women should be screened prenatally for hepatitis B surface antigen (HBsAg) status as part of the standard prenatal labs that are obtained. Perinatally acquired hepatitis B is associated with the highest risk of developing chronic disease in the newborn. A 3-dose hepatitis B vaccine series should be started for pregnant women who have not been vaccinated previously and are at high risk of acquiring the disease, namely those with more than one sex partner during the previous 6 months, those evaluated or treated for a sexually transmitted disease, those with a history of recent or current injection drug use, those having had an HBsAg-positive sex partner, or those living in a household with a contact infected with hepatitis B.

Pneumococcal Disease
Streptococcus pneumoniae is associated with significant morbidity and mortality related to pneumonia, meningitis, and bacteremia. Risk factors for acquiring disease include chronic heart disease, chronic lung disease (which includes asthma), diabetes, cigarette smoking, alcoholism, chronic liver disease, cerebrospinal fluid leaks, cochlear implants, congenital or acquired immunodeficiency, diseases requiring immunosuppressive therapy, sickle cell disease and other hemoglobinopathies, and functional or anatomic asplenia.

Observational studies of PPSV23 vaccine in pregnancy have shown no increases in spontaneous abortion, teratogenicity, or preterm labor, and a randomized trial of pregnant women receiving PPSV23 at 35 weeks of gestation showed no adverse effects. There are insufficient data to recommend routine administration of either PCV15/PCV20 or PPSV23 during pregnancy. The safety of pneumococcal polysaccharide vaccine during the first trimester of pregnancy has not been evaluated, although no adverse consequences have been reported among newborns whose mothers were inadvertently vaccinated early in pregnancy.

Pneumococcal conjugate vaccines (PCV15 and PCV20) appear to be safe when administered during the second or third trimester of pregnancy. The safety of the pneumococcal conjugate vaccines during the first trimester of pregnancy has not been evaluated.

Meningococcal Disease
Meningococcal quadrivalent protein conjugate vaccines are inactivated vaccines and have not been associated with adverse

maternal or fetal outcomes; however, there are no data available on the safety of vaccination with the quadrivalent protein conjugate vaccine during pregnancy. The CDC states that pregnancy should not prevent vaccination with the quadrivalent protein conjugate vaccine in high-risk situations, but the meningococcal B vaccine should be postponed until after pregnancy and breastfeeding unless there is a significant chance for infection.

There are no data available on the use of the pentavalent protein conjugate vaccine during pregnancy.

Polio
Although no adverse effects of inactivated polio vaccine (IPV) have been documented among pregnant women or their fetuses, vaccination of pregnant women should be avoided on theoretical grounds. However, if a pregnant woman is at increased risk for infection and requires immediate protection against polio, IPV can be administered in accordance with the recommended schedules for adults.

Typhoid Fever
No data have been reported on the use of any of the typhoid fever vaccines in pregnant women. No animal studies or controlled studies have been performed.

Japanese Encephalitis
No controlled studies have assessed the safety, immunogenicity, or efficacy of Ixiaro in pregnant women. Preclinical studies of Ixiaro in pregnant rats did not show evidence of harm to the mother or fetus.

Yellow Fever
Pregnancy is a precaution for yellow fever (YF) vaccine administration, compared with most other live vaccines, which are

contraindicated in pregnancy. In areas where YF is endemic, or during outbreaks, the benefits of YF vaccination are likely to far outweigh the risk of potential transmission of vaccine virus to the fetus or infant. If travel is unavoidable, and the risks for YF virus exposure are believed to outweigh the vaccination risks, a pregnant woman should be vaccinated. If the risks for vaccination are believed to outweigh the risks for YF virus exposure, pregnant women should be issued a medical waiver to fulfill health regulations in the various countries. Although no specific data are available, a woman should wait 4 weeks after receiving YF vaccine before conceiving.

Rabies

Because of the potential consequences of inadequately managed rabies exposure, pregnancy is not considered a contraindication to post-exposure prophylaxis. Certain studies have indicated no increased incidence of abortion, premature births, or fetal abnormalities associated with rabies vaccination. If the risk of exposure to rabies is substantial, pre-exposure prophylaxis also might be indicated during pregnancy. Rabies exposure or the diagnosis of rabies in the mother should not be regarded as justification for terminating the pregnancy.

Cholera Vaccine

Live, attenuated oral cholera vaccine is not absorbed systemically following oral administration, and maternal use is not expected to result in fetal exposure to the drug. Breastfeeding is also not expected to result in exposure of the infant to the drug. The vaccine may be considered for use in pregnant women who may be traveling to and/or working in cholera-affected countries, as maternal cholera disease is associated with adverse pregnancy outcomes including fetal death. The vaccine strain may be shed in the stool of the vaccinated mother for at least 7 days, with a potential for transmission of the vaccine strain from the mother to infant during vaginal delivery.

Mpox Vaccine
Currently, no vaccine against mpox is approved for use in pregnancy. Because MVA-BN is a non-replicating, live, attenuated vaccine, there is no theoretical reason for concern about its use in pregnancy. Studies performed in animals did not find any adverse fetal effects.

Dengue Vaccine
The live, attenuated, tetravalent dengue vaccine (CYD-TDV) is licensed for use in the United States and in a number of endemic countries. Despite the risk of obstetric complications in pregnant women due to infection with dengue virus infection, this vaccine is contraindicated for use during pregnancy. In a small study, no increased adverse pregnancy outcomes were identified from inadvertent immunization of women in early pregnancy with CYD-TDV compared with the control group.

Frequently Asked Questions

Is it safe to receive a flu shot during pregnancy and at any specific time in pregnancy?
Yes, flu vaccine can be given at any time in pregnancy. Influenza is particularly dangerous during pregnancy, especially in the later trimesters, and can lead to serious complications and hospitalization. Severe complications can also occur in infants born to mothers with influenza.

If a patient is inadvertently given an MMR vaccine early in an unsuspected pregnancy, should the pregnancy be terminated?
No. There have been no cases of congenital rubella syndrome associated with inadvertent MMR vaccination during pregnancy.

Should a pregnant woman who is traveling to an area of the world where yellow fever is endemic be vaccinated with yellow fever vaccine?
Pregnancy is a precaution for yellow fever (YF) vaccine administration. If travel is unavoidable, and the risks for YF virus exposure (endemic area or during outbreak) are believed to outweigh the vaccination risks, a pregnant woman should be vaccinated.

Should grandparents from out of town be vaccinated with Tdap before visiting their newborn grandchild?
Yes. If they have not been previously vaccinated, they should be vaccinated prior to the visit.

If a pregnant women receives the RSV vaccine, should her infant receive nirsevimab (RSV extended-duration monoclonal antibody) after birth?
No. The CDC recommends that nirsevimab be given to infants younger than age 8 months born during or entering first RSV season if their mother did not receive RSV vaccine, the mother's vaccination status is unknown, or if the infant is born less than 14 days after the mother's vaccination.

PART III

ROUTINE VACCINES FOR VACCINE-PREVENTABLE DISEASES

DIPHTHERIA

Did you know that:

- Abraham Lincoln had four sons, two of whom died from vaccine-preventable infectious diseases. Eddie, Lincoln's second son, died at age 2 years from diphtheria. His third son, Willie, died at age 11 years from typhoid fever.
- The only son of Dr. Abraham Jacobi, who is often referred to as the "father of American Pediatrics," died of diphtheria at age 8 years, a disease of which his father was a recognized authority.
- Historical descriptions of diphtheria (throat membrane, neck swelling, and suffocation) first appeared in ancient Egyptian writings from the second millennium BC.
- In 1921, there were 206,000 cases of diphtheria in the United States, resulting in 15,520 deaths. Twenty percent of children younger than age 5 years died from diphtheria.

Diphtheria is caused by toxigenic strains of the gram-positive, non-spore-forming, nonmotile, pleomorphic bacillus *Corynebacterium diphtheriae*. The disease can have a variety of manifestations, including respiratory tract diphtheria, which presents as membranous nasopharyngitis or obstructive laryngotracheitis. Onset of the disease is abrupt, with sore throat; mild pharyngeal injection; and the development of a gray membrane on one or both tonsils with extension to the tonsillar pillars, uvula, soft palate, oropharynx, and nasopharynx with a bloody nasal discharge. Involvement of the larynx and bronchi presents with symptoms of hoarseness, dyspnea, respiratory stridor, a brassy cough, cyanosis, retractions, and respiratory distress. Diphtheria may also present as cutaneous, vaginal, conjunctival, or otic disease; and as mycotic aneurysms, septic arthritis, and osteomyelitis. Local infections are associated with low-grade fever, malaise, and the gradual onset of manifestations over 1 to 2 days. Extensive neck swelling with cervical lymphadenitis (bull neck) is a sign of severe disease that occurs more often in persons who are unimmunized or inadequately immunized. Diphtheria remains endemic in the former Soviet Union, Africa, Latin America, Haiti, Asia, the Middle East, and areas of Europe where childhood immunization coverage with diphtheria toxoid-containing vaccines is suboptimal.

Life-threatening complications of respiratory diphtheria include upper airway obstruction caused by extensive membrane formation; myocarditis (detected in up to two-thirds of patients), which is often associated with varying degrees of heart block and myocardial dysfunction; cranial and peripheral neuropathies; and palatal palsy associated with pharyngeal diphtheria characterized by nasal speech.

Transmission

Humans are the sole reservoir of *C. diphtheriae*. Organisms are spread by intimate contact with airborne respiratory tract droplets from persons with active infection or carriers and by contact with exudates from infected skin lesions. People who travel to areas where diphtheria is endemic or people who come into contact with infected travelers from such areas are at increased risk of being infected with the organism.

Incubation Period

The incubation period is 2 to 7 days (range: 1–10 days).

Prevention

Post-exposure

a. Persons who have diphtheria disease and are in the convalescent stage of their disease should receive a dose of a diphtheria toxoid-containing vaccine because clinical infection does not always induce adequate levels of antitoxin.

b. Close contacts of persons with diphtheria disease, regardless of their immunization status, should receive antibiotic prophylaxis with erythromycin (40–50 mg/kg per day for 7–10 days, max 1 gram per day) or single intramuscular injection of penicillin G benzathine (600,000 U for children weighing <30 kg and 1.2 million U for children weighing ≥30 kg and for adults), *and* should receive a dose of a diphtheria toxoid-containing vaccine.

Pre-exposure
   a. Diphtheria toxoid-containing vaccines—type of vaccine varies by age.
      i. For infants and children from 6 weeks to 7 years of age—five intramuscular doses of DTaP vaccines are recommended, beginning at 6 to 8 weeks of age. Recommended doses are given at 2 months, 4 months, 6 months, 12 to 18 months, and 4 to 6 years of age in the United States.
      ii. For persons older than 7 years of age—an intramuscular dose of Td vaccine should be administered if immunization against diphtheria or tetanus is indicated. A dose of Tdap vaccine (contains acellular pertussis) may also be given if a previous dose has not been received. Booster doses of Tdap are recommended every 8 to 10 years.

Duration of Immunity

Approximately 10 years.

Contraindications and Precautions to Diphtheria-Containing Vaccines

Contraindications
Severe immediate allergic reaction (e.g., anaphylaxis) to a prior dose of tetanus and diphtheria toxoid-containing vaccines (e.g., DTaP, Tdap, Td) is a contraindication to further doses.

Precautions
1. Moderate or severe acute illness with or without fever
2. Guillain–Barré syndrome within 6 weeks after a previous dose of tetanus toxoid-containing vaccine
3. History of Arthus-type hypersensitivity reactions after a previous dose of tetanus or diphtheria toxoid-containing vaccine; defer vaccination until at least 10 years have elapsed since the last tetanus toxoid-containing vaccine.

Frequently Asked Questions

Diphtheria is rare in the United States. Are there countries where diphtheria is still prevalent?
Yes, there are countries where diphtheria is still prevalent and poses a risk. These include countries in Asia (the Philippines, Nepal, Indonesia, Bangladesh, Vietnam, Laos), Africa, the Middle East (Pakistan, India, Afghanistan), the countries of the former Soviet Union (Russia, Ukraine, the Baltic States, and Georgia), Latin America (Venezuela), the South Pacific, Eastern Europe, Haiti, and the Dominican Republic. Persons traveling to these countries should ensure that they are up to date with their diphtheria toxoid vaccination status.

Who is at risk of acquiring diphtheria?
Persons, especially children, who are not immunized or who did not receive adequate immunization are at the highest risk. Diphtheria is most common in areas where people live in crowded conditions with poor sanitation.

If a person is infected with diphtheria, how long are they contagious and able to spread disease to others?
Untreated people who are infected with the diphtheria organism can be contagious for up to 2 weeks but rarely more than 4 weeks. If treated with appropriate antibiotics, the contagious period can be limited to less than 4 days.

What are the potential consequences of not being treated for diphtheria?
If diphtheria goes untreated, serious complications such as upper airway obstruction, paralysis and cranial and peripheral neuropathies, encephalitis, cerebral infarction, myocarditis, heart failure with heart block, and renal failure may occur. Death occurs in approximately 5% to 10% of all cases.

Does past infection with diphtheria make a person immune to the disease?
Unfortunately, a person who recovers from diphtheria does not reliably develop lasting immunity to the disease and needs diphtheria-containing vaccines to develop protective immunity.

TETANUS

Did you know that:

- John Augustus Roebling, the architect of the Brooklyn Bridge, died from tetanus after his leg was crushed by a ferryboat while working on the bridge.
- John Thoreau, brother of famous American writer and transcendentalist Henry David Thoreau, died from tetanus after cutting himself shaving.

- Tetanus is called "lockjaw" because one of the first symptoms of the disease is severe muscle spasms of the jaw muscles preventing opening of the mouth.

Tetanus (lockjaw) occurs worldwide and is more common in warmer climates and during warmer months. It is caused by neurotoxin produced by the anaerobic, spore-forming, gram-positive bacterium *Clostridium tetani*, which is a normal inhabitant of soil, animal and human intestines, and is ubiquitous in the environment. The organism multiplies in wounds and elaborates toxins in the presence of anaerobic conditions. Contaminated wounds, especially wounds with devitalized tissue and deep-puncture trauma, are at greatest risk (including frostbite). Neonatal tetanus is common in many developing countries in which pregnant women are not immunized appropriately against tetanus and nonsterile umbilical cord care practices are followed.

Tetanus has four clinical forms:

1. Generalized tetanus (lockjaw) is a neurologic disease manifesting as severe muscle spasms, including trismus (jaw muscle spasms or lockjaw), risus sardonicus (facial muscle spasms resulting in a sardonic grin), and opisthotonus (severe spasm and hyperextension of the neck and spine). Onset is gradual, occurring over 1 to 7 days, and symptoms rapidly progress to severe generalized muscle spasms, which are made worse by any external stimuli. Severe spasms persist for 1 or more weeks and subside over several weeks in persons who survive. Other symptoms include fever, diaphoresis, tachycardia, and elevated blood pressure associated with sympathetic overactivity.

2. Local tetanus manifests as local muscle spasms in areas contiguous to a contaminated wound that very often progresses to generalized tetanus.
3. Neonatal tetanus is a form of generalized tetanus occurring in newborn infants who lack protective passive immunity because their mothers are not immunized. Neonates present with generalized weakness and failure to nurse followed by apnea, rigidity, and spasms. Mortality rate exceeds 90%, and developmental delays are common among survivors.
4. Cephalic tetanus is a dysfunction of cranial nerves associated with infected wounds on the head and neck. Cephalic tetanus can progress to generalized tetanus.

Transmission

Contamination of wounds. The vegetative form of *C. tetani* produces a potent plasmid-encoded exotoxin (tetanospasmin), which binds to gangliosides at the myoneuronal junction of skeletal muscle and on neuronal membranes in the spinal cord, blocking inhibitory impulses to motor neurons.

Incubation Period

The incubation period is 3 to 21 days, with the majority of cases occurring within 8 days. Shorter incubation periods are associated with more heavily contaminated wounds, more severe disease, and a worse prognosis. For neonatal tetanus, symptoms appear on average 7 days after birth (range: 4–14 days).

Prevention

Post-exposure

a. Tetanus toxoid-containing vaccine with or without human tetanus immune globulin (TIG) in the management of wounds depends on the type of wound and the immunization history with tetanus toxoid (Table 8). DTaP is used for children younger than 7 years of age. Tdap is preferred over Td for underimmunized persons 7 years of age or older who have not received a prior dose of Tdap.

When an infant is born outside the hospital and the umbilical cord is likely contaminated (e.g., cut with nonsterile equipment), the

Table 8 MANAGEMENT OF WOUNDS DEPENDING ON WOUND TYPE AND TETANUS TOXOID IMMUNIZATION HISTORY

Number of Tetanus Toxoid Doses	Clean, Minor Wounds DTaP/Tdap/Td	TIG	All Other Wounds DTaP/Tdap/Td	TIG
≤3 or unknown	Yes	No	Yes	Yes
3 or more	**No** if <10 years since last tetanus-containing vaccine	No	**No** if <5 years since last tetanus-containing vaccine	No
	Yes if >10 years since last tetanus-containing vaccine	No	**Yes** if ≥5 years since last tetanus-containing vaccine	No

maternal history of tetanus immunization should be confirmed. If the mother's tetanus immunization status is unknown and she is unlikely to have been immunized, TIG should be administered to the neonate unless the maternal tetanus serostatus can be confirmed quickly.

For infants younger than 6 months of age who have not received a full 3-dose primary series of tetanus toxoid-containing vaccine, decisions on the need for TIG with wound care should be based on the mother's tetanus toxoid immunization history at the time of delivery.

Pre-exposure
- a. Active immunization with tetanus toxoid-containing vaccine is recommended for persons of all ages. Tetanus immunization is administered with diphtheria toxoid-containing vaccines (e.g., Td) or with diphtheria toxoid- and acellular pertussis-containing vaccines (e.g., DTaP, Tdap)—the type of vaccine varies by age. Vaccines are administered intramuscularly.
    - i. For infants and children from 6 weeks up to 7 years of age—five intramuscular doses of DTaP vaccines are recommended, beginning at 6 to 8 weeks of age. Recommended doses are given at 2 months, 4 months, 6 months, 12 to 18 months and 4 to 6 years of age in the United States.
    - ii. For persons ≥7 years of age—an intramuscular dose of Td vaccine is given if immunization against diphtheria or tetanus is needed. A dose of Tdap vaccine (contains acellular pertussis) may also be given if a previous dose has not been received. Booster doses of Tdap are recommended every 8 to 10 years.

Duration of Immunity

Approximately 10 years.

Contraindications and Precautions

Contraindications

Severe immediate allergic reaction (e.g., anaphylaxis) to a prior dose of tetanus and diphtheria toxoid-containing vaccines (e.g. DTaP, Tdap, Td) is a contraindication to further doses.

Precautions
1. Moderate or severe acute illness with or without fever
2. Guillain–Barré syndrome within 6 weeks after a previous dose of tetanus toxoid-containing vaccine
3. History of Arthus-type hypersensitivity reactions after a previous dose of tetanus or diphtheria toxoid-containing vaccine; defer vaccination until at least 10 years have elapsed since the last tetanus toxoid-containing vaccine.

Frequently Asked Questions

If a person sustains a puncture wound or laceration that is tetanus prone (e.g., wounds contaminated with soil or fecal material), does the person need to receive tetanus wound management the day that the injury occurred or can this wait for 48 to 72 hours?

Puncture wounds should be attended to as soon as possible. The decision to delay a booster dose of tetanus toxoid-containing vaccine following an injury should be based on the type of injury and likelihood that the person is susceptible to tetanus. The more likely the person is to be susceptible (e.g., unvaccinated or incompletely vaccinated against tetanus), the more quickly the tetanus prophylaxis (TIG and Tdap/Td) should be administered.

When should tetanus immune globulin (TIG) be administered as part of wound management?
TIG is recommended for any wound other than a clean minor wound if the person's vaccination history is either unknown or they have had less than a complete series of 3 doses of Td vaccine. TIG should be given as soon as possible after the injury.

How long after a wound occurs is TIG no longer recommended?
For a person who has been vaccinated but is not up to date, there is little benefit in giving TIG more than 1 week after the injury. For a person who is completely vaccinated, this interval can be increased to up to day 21 post-injury period.

If an adult patient states that they had tetanus infection as a child but does not know if they have ever received any tetanus-containing vaccines, should this patient be immunized with a tetanus-containing vaccine as part of routine health maintenance?
A history of tetanus disease is not a reason to avoid using tetanus-containing vaccines. Tetanus disease does not produce immunity because only a very small amount of toxin is needed to produce disease. If the patient has no other contraindications, they should receive a tetanus-containing vaccine now. If they have no documentation of prior tetanus vaccination, they should complete a 3-dose series with Tdap, followed by a dose of Td 4 to 8 weeks later, and a dose of Td 6 to 12 months after the last Td dose.

Should an adult patient who previously received a Tdap vaccine receive another Tdap vaccine after a bone marrow transplant?
Yes. A dose of Tdap vaccine 6 months after a bone marrow transplant is appropriate.

Can Tdap and RhoGam (anti-Rho[D]) immunoglobulin be given at the same prenatal visit?
Yes. Tdap is an inactivated vaccine and may be given at the same prenatal visit with RhoGam.

PERTUSSIS

Did you know that:

- George Washington Carver (American botanist and inventor), Dolly Madison (wife of U.S. President James Madison), and Shah Mohammed Reza Pahlavi (the Shah of Iran) all suffered from bouts of pertussis.
- Pertussis is also known as "whooping cough" because of the "whooping" sound that is made when gasping for air after a fit of coughing.
- Coughing fits due to pertussis infection can last for up to 10 weeks or more; this disease has been called the "cough of 100 days."

Pertussis (whooping cough) is caused by the gram-negative organism *Bordetella pertussis*. Humans are the only known hosts of the organism. It continues to be a major public health problem in all age groups and is the cause of major epidemics worldwide. Cases occur year-round. The incidence of disease in the adolescent and adult populations has significantly increased during the past several decades primarily due to waning of both vaccine and naturally induced immunity and increased disease awareness associated with the use of respiratory pathogen panel testing which contains pertussis as a pathogen in the panel. Neither natural infection nor immunization provides lifelong immunity. Older children, adolescents, and adults serve as the major reservoirs of pertussis disease in the community. Young infants, especially those younger than 3 months of age, are at the greatest risk for morbidity and mortality from disease. Since 1990, 93% to 100% of pertussis deaths in the United States have occurred in this very young infant population. The CDC, AAP, IOM, American Academy of Family Physicians (AAFP), and ACOG all strongly support immunization of pregnant women and a "cocoon strategy" to protect these young infants. This strategy focuses on the targeted immunization of older children, adolescents, and adults who either live in the household or who are close contacts of these young infants to prevent these individuals from getting pertussis disease and giving it to the young infants. This should include all adolescents and adults, including persons older than age 65 years, grandparents, relatives, friends, nannies, babysitters, day care providers, and housekeepers.

Pertussis disease consists of three stages, and severity of disease ranges from very mild, atypical disease to severe classic pertussis (Table 9):

Stage 1: Catarrhal stage—symptoms are mild and include rhinorrhea with no pharyngitis, mild conjunctival injection, low-grade fever or no fever, and mild cough. This stage lasts for 2 weeks.

Table 9 CLINICAL SIGNS AND SYMPTOMS OF PERTUSSIS IN ADOLESCENTS AND ADULTS[a]

	Center Age Group over Adolescents and Adults	
Clinical Characteristic	Adolescents (%) (10–19 Years)	Adults (%) (≥20 Years)
Paroxysms of cough	82.5 (82–83)	87 (33–100)
Inspiratory whoop	50 (30–67)	74 (7–82)
Apnea	46 (19–86)	85 (29–87)
Cyanosis	6–15	9–12
Posttussive emesis	56 (45–71)	50 (17–70)
Hospitalization	1.4–7.5	3.5–5.7

[a]Based on a compilation of eight different studies.

Stage 2: Paroxysmal stage—symptoms include paroxysms of cough, posttussive emesis, inspiratory whooping, apnea, and cyanosis. Symptoms may be milder in individuals who have received immunization in the past and in the adolescent and adult populations. This stage lasts for 6 weeks.

Stage 3: Convalescent stage—coughing paroxysms and other symptoms become less frequent and intense. This stage lasts for 4 to 6 weeks.

Persons with pertussis may be ill for 3 or 4 months from onset of cough. Any intercurrent viral illness will exacerbate cough illness. Treatment with antibiotic therapy is effective in preventing transmission of the organism but does not have an impact on the duration of the cough. Negative quality of life has a very large impact on adolescent and adult patients with pertussis. The vast majority are unable to sleep, go to work, attend school, or eat or drink normally during their illness.

Pertussis should be included in the differential of all adolescents and adults presenting for evaluation of a persistent cough illness lasting 2 weeks or more.

Infants, especially those younger than 3 months of age, who are unimmunized or who have received only the first of their primary immunizations, are at the greatest risk for complications, hospitalizations, and deaths due to pertussis disease. Apnea alone or apnea associated with very mild cough may be the only presenting symptom of pertussis in this age group. Complications seen among infants include pneumonia (22%), seizures (2%), encephalopathy (<0.5%), pulmonary hypertension, hernia, subdural bleeding, conjunctival bleeding, and death.

Complications in Children, Adolescents, and Adults

Complications include pneumonia (1.9% in patients <30 years of age, 5-9% in older patients), seizures (0.3%), encephalopathy (0.1%), urinary incontinence (4% of adults, 35% of women >50 years), pneumothorax, inguinal hernia, aspiration pneumonia, fractured ribs, hearing loss, syncope, subconjunctival hemorrhages, carotid artery dissection, and intracranial bleeding. Incidence of complications increases with age.

Antibiotics used in the treatment of cases and chemoprophylaxis of close contacts are shown in Table 10.

Table 10 ANTIBIOTIC TREATMENT AND PROPHYLACTIC REGIMENS FOR PERTUSSIS

Antibiotic	Dosage	Comments
Erythromycin estolate or erythromycin ethylsuccinate	40–50 mg/kg/day (max 2 grams/day) PO divided q 6–8 hours × 14 days	Contraindicated in infants <6 weeks of age due to increased risk for pyloric stenosis
Azithromycin	10 mg/kg/day × 5 days (infants <6 months); 10 mg/kg on day 1 (max 500 mg/day) then 5 mg/kg per day on days 2–5 (max 250 mg/day)	*Drug of choice for all age groups*
Clarithromycin	15–20 mg/kg/day (max 1 gram/day) q 8–12 hours × 7–10 days	—
Trimethoprim-sulfamethoxazole (TMP/SMX)	8 mg TMP/40 mg SMX per kg/day (max 320 mg TMP/1,600 mg SMX/day) in 2 divided doses × 14 days	Drug of choice for patients who cannot tolerate the macrolide antibiotics or who are allergic to the macrolide antibiotics

Persons who should receive chemoprophylaxis include the following:

- All household contacts **regardless of age and immunization status**
- Other close contacts regardless of age and immunization status defined by the CDC as:

- Anyone who has had face-to-face contact or shared a confined space for a prolonged period of time (>1 hour) with an infected individua
- Persons who have direct contact with respiratory, oral, or nasal secretions from a symptomatic patient (e.g., cough, sneeze, sharing food and eating utensils, mouth-to-mouth resuscitation, or performing a medical examination of the mouth, nose, and throat)

Transmission

Close contact with cases via aerosolized respiratory droplets. Persons are infectious beginning with the first day of cough and if untreated can continue to transmit the organism for up to 3 weeks after onset of illness.

Prevention

Post-exposure
  a. Antibiotic chemoprophylaxis for all household and close contacts as above in addition to pertussis-containing vaccines.
  b. Pertussis-containing vaccines are recommended for all unimmunized or incompletely immunized household and close contacts. Pertussis immunization is administered with diphtheria and tetanus toxoid-containing vaccines (e.g., DTaP, Tdap)—type of vaccine varies by age. Vaccines are administered intramuscularly. DTaP is used for children younger than 7 years of age. Tdap is used for unimmunized or incompletely immunized persons older than 7 years of age who have not received a prior dose of Tdap.

Pre-exposure
PERTUSSIS-CONTAINING VACCINES
i. For infants and children from 6 weeks up to 7 years of age—5 intramuscular doses of DTaP vaccines are recommended, beginning at 6 to 8 weeks of age. Recommended doses are given at 2 months, 4 months, 6 months, 12 to 18 months, and 4 to 6 years of age.
ii. For persons ≥7 years of age—an intramuscular dose of Tdap vaccine is given if immunization against pertussis is needed and if a previous dose has not been received. Tdap boosters are recommended every 8 to 10 years, except in the case of pregnant women.
iii. It is recommended that pregnant women receive a dose of Tdap vaccine after 20 weeks of gestation (during the late second or third trimesters of pregnancy) for *each* pregnancy, regardless of prior immunization status or time interval since previous Tdap dose.
iv. If a woman is unable to receive a dose of Tdap during pregnancy, postpartum administration of a dose of Tdap is a viable option for women who have not received a previous Tdap dose. The dose should be given as soon as possible after delivery but before hospital discharge.
v. Tdap vaccine is recommended for all adolescents starting at 11 or 12 years of age and all adults **regardless** of the interval from the last dose of Td vaccine.
vi. Tdap vaccine is strongly recommended for all health care workers who have any direct patient contact either in a hospital or clinic setting **regardless** of the interval from the last dose of Td vaccine.

Duration of Immunity

The duration is 3 to 5 years after last dose of pertussis-containing vaccine. Immunity is at best 10 years after natural infection.

Contraindications and Precautions

Contraindications
1. Encephalopathy (e.g., coma, decreased level of consciousness, prolonged seizures) not attributable to another identifiable cause within 7 days of administration of a previous dose of DTP or DTaP (for DTaP); or a previous dose of DTP, DTaP, or Tdap (Tdap).
2. Severe immediate allergic reaction (e.g., anaphylaxis) to a prior dose of vaccine or to a vaccine component

Precautions
1. Moderate or severe acute illness with or without fever
2. Guillain–Barré syndrome within 6 weeks after a previous dose of tetanus toxoid-containing vaccine
3. Progressive or unstable neurologic disorder (including infantile spasms for DTaP), uncontrolled seizures, or progressive encephalopathy until a treatment regimen has been established and the condition has stabilized
4. For DTaP only
   a. Temperature of 105°F or higher (40.5°C or higher) within 48 hours after vaccination with a previous dose of DTP/DTaP
   b. Collapse or shocklike state (i.e., hypotonic hyporesponsive episode) within 48 hours after receiving a previous dose of DTP/DTaP

c. Seizure within 3 days after receiving a previous dose of DTP/DTaP
d. Persistent, inconsolable crying lasting 3 or more hours within 48 hours after receiving a previous dose of DTP/DTaP

Frequently Asked Questions

If a person (infant, child, or adult) has had a documented case of pertussis, can they get the disease again?
Reinfection is uncommon, but it does occur. Symptoms with reinfection may present as only a persistent cough with little else.

If a person (infant, child, adolescent, or adult) has had pertussis disease, should they still be vaccinated with a pertussis-containing vaccine?
Yes. All persons who have a history of pertussis disease generally should receive pertussis-containing vaccines (DTaP or Tdap) according to the routine schedule. This is recommended because the amount and duration of protection induced by pertussis disease are unknown and because the diagnosis of pertussis can be difficult to confirm.

Which health care workers (HCWs) should be vaccinated against pertussis with tetanus–diphtheria–acellular pertussis (Tdap) vaccine?
The CDC recommends that all HCWs, regardless of age, should receive a dose of Tdap as soon as feasible if they have not previously received Tdap and regardless of the time since their last Td vaccine.

If an HCW has been vaccinated with Tdap vaccine and then has a significant exposure to someone with pertussis, does the vaccinated HCW need to be treated with prophylactic antibiotics or are they considered immune to the disease?
All HCWs who have a significant exposure to pertussis disease should receive antibiotic prophylaxis regardless of their immunization status. The effectiveness of Tdap in preventing pertussis in the health care setting is currently unknown. Until studies can be performed that define the optimal management of exposed vaccinated HCWs, the CDC's post-exposure prophylaxis protocol for pertussis exposure should be followed.

How many doses of pediatric diphtheria–tetanus–acellular pertussis (DTaP) vaccine does an infant need before they are protected from pertussis?
Vaccine efficacy following 3 doses of pediatric DTaP vaccine is 80% to 85%. Information regarding efficacy after 1 or 2 doses is limited, but efficacy is most likely lower. In order to protect the infant against pertussis prior to them receiving their 3-dose primary DTaP vaccine series, it is important that all people who live in the household with the infant and all those who provide care to them (e.g., babysitters, nannies, au pairs, and day care providers) be protected against pertussis. It is recommended that these individuals receive a dose of adolescent/adult Tdap if they have not already done so.

What should be done in the situation in which a 4-month-old infant inadvertently received a dose of adolescent/adult Tdap instead of pediatric DTaP?
If Tdap is inadvertently administered to a child younger than 7 years of age, it should *not* be counted as valid for the first,

second, or third dose of DTaP (primary vaccine series). The dose should be repeated with a dose of DTaP, and the routine vaccination schedule should be followed. If the dose of Tdap was administered for the fourth or fifth booster dose, the Tdap dose can be counted as valid.

What should be done in the situation in which a 10-year-old child inadvertently received a dose of DTaP instead of Tdap?
DTaP given to patients aged 7 years or older can be counted as valid for the Tdap dose.

In the situation in which an 18-year-old patient received only 2 doses of DTP (whole cell pertussis vaccine) at 2 months and 4 months of age after developing persistent crying and a temperature of 105°F following the second dose of DTP vaccine, is it safe to give this patient a dose of Tdap vaccine?
Yes, it is safe to give a dose of Tdap vaccine. Many of the precautions to DTP and DTaP (e.g., temperature of 105°F or higher, persistent crying lasting 3 hours of longer, seizure with or without fever, and hyporesponsive or shocklike state) do not apply to the Tdap vaccine.

A 2-month-old received her first dose of DTaP vaccine and then developed inconsolable crying for more than 3 hours. Should the infant receive additional doses of DTaP or should they be given DT vaccine?
Persistent crying following DTaP has been observed much less frequently than it was following the use of DTP (whole cell pertussis) vaccine. When it occurs following DTaP, it is considered

a precaution. If the benefit of the pertussis vaccine exceeds the risk of persistent crying (which in itself is benign), one can administer additional doses of DTaP. Many providers choose to administer pertussis-containing vaccine if this is the only precaution the infant has experienced. The health care provider and the parent(s) will need to make this judgment.

Is there an upper age limit for Tdap administration?
There is *no* upper age limit for Tdap vaccination. A dose of Tdap is recommended for all adults regardless of age, with booster doses recommended every 8 to 10 years.

Which adults should be vaccinated with a Tdap vaccine?
The CDC recommends that *all* adults aged 19 years or older receive a dose of Tdap vaccine regardless of the interval since the last tetanus or diphtheria toxoid-containing vaccine (e.g., Td). A booster dose of Tdap is recommended every 8 to 10 years.

What should be done in the situation in which a patient remembers receiving a "tetanus booster" several years ago at a convenient care clinic but no vaccination record is available and the patient does not remember if he received Td or Tdap? The patient's wife is 37 weeks pregnant. Can the patient receive a dose of Tdap vaccine as a way to protect their soon-to-be-born child against pertussis?
Yes. If vaccination is indicated and there is a lack of vaccine documentation, a dose of Tdap can be given to the patient.

If a pregnant woman got a dose of Td during pregnancy, how soon can she get her dose of Tdap?

She should have been given Tdap rather than Td; however, she can receive her Tdap *at any interval* since the Td dose was given, preferably between 27 and 36 weeks of gestation.

If a woman received a dose of Tdap early in her pregnancy (e.g., in her first trimester), should she get another dose in the third trimester?
No, it is not recommended to give another dose of Tdap. The optimal timing for Tdap administration in pregnancy is between 27 and 36 weeks of gestation because of the favorable transplacental antibody kinetics. Tdap may be administered at any time during pregnancy, but vaccination during the third trimester would provide the highest concentration of maternal antibodies to be transferred.

Should fathers and other family members receive a Tdap booster each time there is a pregnancy in the family to boost the cocoon effect to protect the newborn from pertussis?
At this time, the CDC does not recommend additional doses of Tdap vaccine for fathers, other family members, or caregivers. The recommendation for a dose of Tdap with each pregnancy only applies to the pregnant woman.

Can Tdap vaccine be given to breastfeeding mothers?
Yes. Women who have never received Tdap and who did not receive it during pregnancy should receive it immediately postpartum or as soon as feasibly possible. Breastfeeding does not decrease the immune response to routine childhood vaccine.

My practice is seeing a number of patients who are refugees or who have immigrated from other countries. What vaccine schedule should be used to vaccinate children,

adolescents, or adults who have never received the primary series of tetanus toxoid-containing vaccines?
Children 7 years of age or older and adolescents and adults who have never received tetanus-containing vaccines or whose vaccination history is unknown should receive a 3-dose vaccine series. The CDC recommends Tdap at 0 and Td at 4 weeks and at least 6 months. Tdap can be substituted for only one of the 3 Td doses in the series, preferably the first. The amount of protection provided by a single dose of Tdap in a person who has not previously received pertussis vaccine is not known. Following the primary series, booster doses of Td should be given every 10 years.

If a child has already received 5 appropriately spaced doses of DTaP (6-month intervals between doses 3 and 4 and doses 4 and 5) by their fourth birthday, should a booster dose be given after the fourth birthday?
As a rule, a child should receive no more than 4 doses of DTaP before 4 years of age. The CDC recommends that a dose of DTaP be given at 4 to 6 years of age. Many states have school immunization laws which require that at least 1 dose of DTP/DTaP be given on or after the fourth birthday. This dose is important to boost immunity to pertussis.

INFLUENZA

Did you know that:

- The word "influenza" comes from the Italian *influentia* because it was believed that the influence of the planets,

moon, and stars caused the flu—for only such universal influence could explain such sudden and widespread illness.
- Martin van Buren, the eighth president of the United States; Benjamin Harrison, the twenty-third president of the United States; Juan Peron, the former president of Argentina; Shoghi Effendi, the Guardian and appointed head of the Baha'i faith; and Sir William Osler, physician, educator, and medical philosopher, all died from severe influenza infections.
- The Spanish influenza pandemic of 1918 killed between 20 million and 40 million people, which is more than the number who died during World War I. More people died in 1 year from this pandemic than in 4 years of the Black Death (bubonic plague) from 1347 to 1351. The death rate for 15- to 34-year-olds of influenza and pneumonia was 20 times higher in 1918 than in previous years. People were struck with illness on the street and died rapid deaths— "people on their way to work suddenly developing the flu and dying within hours."
- The 2009 influenza A H1N1 pandemic influenza virus was found to be transmitted back and forth between infected sick pigs to humans and from infected humans to the pigs they were caring for. The main risk of this human-to-animal infection is that a new reassortant virus could emerge from pigs co-infected by the pandemic virus and by another swine virus. This could lead potentially to a "new" virus with possible increased severity.

Influenza causes annual epidemics during the winter months, with up to 20% of the U.S. population becoming ill with influenza A or B viruses. Children are the most likely to acquire and transmit infection given that they are able to shed virus at very high titers and for prolonged periods of time (≥10 days). Up to 40% of healthy children become ill with influenza each year. However, the populations with the highest rates of serious disease, complications, and deaths are persons 65 years of age or older, children younger than 2 years of age, pregnant women, and persons of any age with underlying medical conditions. Each year, complications from influenza are responsible for more than 200,000 hospitalizations and an average of 36,000 deaths, with greater than 50% of the hospitalizations and 90% of the deaths occurring in persons 65 years of age or older. On a societal level, influenza is an extraordinarily expensive disease, with an average of $10 billion being spent each year on health care and work-loss costs.

The clinical presentation of influenza differs by age. The typical symptoms of the sudden onset of fever accompanied by chills or rigors, headache, malaise, diffuse myalgia, nonproductive cough, sore throat, nasal congestion, and rhinorrhea are seen most commonly in the adolescent and adult populations. Children more commonly have fever, nonproductive cough, rhinitis, nasal congestion, nausea, vomiting, abdominal pain, and diarrhea. Symptoms in the elderly population are very nonspecific, with cough and malaise being the most common. Symptoms in all age groups usually resolve after 3 to 7 days; however, cough and malaise may persist for more than 2 weeks.

Persons at increased risk for influenza complications:

- Children 6 to 59 months of age
- Adults 50 years of age or older (especially persons 65 years of age or older)
- Pregnant women and those up to 2 weeks after the end of pregnancy

- Adults and children with chronic pulmonary (including asthma), renal, cardiovascular, hepatic, neurologic, hematologic, or metabolic disorders
- Immunosuppressed patients (immunosuppressive medications, HIV infection)
- Residents in long-term care facilities (of any age)
- Health care personnel
- Morbidly obese people (body mass index ≥40 kg/m^2)
- Household contacts and caregivers of children younger than 5 years of age (especially those younger than 6 months of age) and adults 50 years of age or older
- Children and adolescents (6 months to 18 years) receiving long-term aspirin therapy
- People from certain ethnic and ethnic minority groups are at increased risk for hospitalization with influenza, including non-Hispanic Black persons, Latino or Hispanic persons, and American Indian and Alaskan Native persons.

Immunization rates for all these at-risk populations are well below the levels recommended by the Healthy People 2030 goals.

Complications of Influenza in the Adult Population

These complications include primary influenza pneumonia and/or secondary bacterial pneumonia may be especially severe in pregnant women; exacerbation of underlying pulmonary or cardiac disease; encephalitis; myositis; myocarditis; pericarditis; transverse myelitis; and Guillain–Barré syndrome. Complications of influenza in the pediatric population include acute otitis media; bronchiolitis; laryngotracheobronchitis;

bacterial pneumonia, which may be necrotizing and is most often due to *Staphylococcus aureus* and *Streptococcus pneumoniae*; encephalitis and encephalopathy, which may be necrotizing; dehydration with severe hypotension; respiratory failure; myositis; and transverse myelitis.

Influenza can be particularly severe in pregnant women. The risk of hospitalization for heart and lung problems is more than fourfold higher in pregnant women compared to nonpregnant women, and the risk increases exponentially as pregnancy progresses. This risk is further increased in pregnant women who have asthma. For example, pregnant women infected with the 2009 H1N1 influenza virus were at very high risk for severe or fatal illness and were at significantly increased risk for fetal death, spontaneous abortions, and preterm delivery. In 2009, pregnant women represented 1% of the U.S. population but accounted for 5% of the U.S. deaths from H1N1 disease. More than 91% of the deaths occurred in women in their second and third trimesters of pregnancy.

Transmission

Person-to-person by respiratory droplets or by direct contact with articles contaminated with nasopharyngeal secretions via coughing and sneezing.

Incubation Period

Incubation period is 1 to 4 days (average 2 days). Adults are infectious from the day before symptoms begin through 5 days after illness onset. Children are infectious for several days before onset of symptoms through 10 days or more after illness onset.

Prevention

Post-exposure

a. Influenza vaccine is the primary means of protecting persons against influenza disease and its complications, and it can be administered at any time during influenza season, even when the virus is actively circulating in the community. Vaccines are quadrivalent. Quadrivalent influenza vaccine (containing two influenza A strains and two influenza B strains) became available beginning in the 2013–2014 influenza season. Injectable and intranasal formations are available for this vaccine.

b. Chemoprophylaxis with influenza antiviral drugs is an adjunctive measure, *not* a substitute, for immunization. It may be used in certain situations in order to control and prevent influenza disease. Situations in which chemoprophylaxis may be considered include the following:

- Protection of unimmunized high-risk children or adults or children or adults who were immunized less than 2 weeks before influenza circulation in the community
- Protection of children and adults at increased risk of severe infection or complications, such as high-risk populations for whom the vaccine is contraindicated
- Protection of unimmunized close contacts of persons at high risk
- Protection of immunocompromised persons who may not respond to vaccine
- Control of influenza outbreaks in a closed setting, such as an institution with unimmunized high-risk persons
- Protection of immunized high-risk persons if the vaccine strain poorly matches circulating influenza strains

Oseltamivir (oral), baloxavir (oral), or zanamivir (inhaled) are the recommended oral antiviral agents. Peramivir (IV) is another agent that may be used.

Pre-exposure
a. Influenza vaccine—there are several different formulations of the vaccine and methods of administration that are available.

Influenza Vaccines—United States, 2023–2024 Influenza Season. Vaccines for 2024–2025 Influenza Season are Trivalent.

- Inactivated influenza vaccine, quadrivalent egg-based (IIV4e), standard dose
  - Afluria Quadrivalent
  - Fluarix Quadrivalent
  - FluLaval Quadrivalent
  - Fluzone Quadrivalent
- Inactivated influenza vaccine, quadrivalent cell culture–based (ccIIV), standard dose
  - Flucelvax Quadrivalent
- Inactivated influenza vaccine, quadrivalent (IIV4), high dose
  - Fluzone High-Dose
- Inactivated influenza vaccine, quadrivalent egg-based adjuvanted with MF59 (aIIV4)
  - Fluad Quadrivalent
- Recombinant influenza vaccine (RIV4), standard dose
  - FluBlok
- Live, attenuated influenza vaccine, quadrivalent (LAIV4)

- FluMist Quadrivalent
  i. Quadrivalent inactivated influenza vaccine (IIV4)—given as intramuscular injection to any person 6 months of age or older. ACOG strongly recommends that *all* women who will be pregnant during influenza season receive a dose of inactivated influenza vaccine—IIV4 or IIV3. The vaccine may be given during any trimester of pregnancy. Contraindication: severe anaphylactic reaction to any vaccine component, including egg protein, or after previous dose of any influenza vaccine. Precautions: moderate to severe acute illness with or without fever; history of Guillain–Barré syndrome within 6 weeks of receipt of influenza vaccine.
  ii. Quadrivalent inactivated influenza vaccine (IIV4)—high-dose—given as intramuscular injection—this vaccine contains four times the amount of influenza antigen in standard-dose influenza vaccine. It stimulates older individuals to produce higher levels of antibody and provides enhanced protection against influenza illness. It is associated with a higher risk of local injection site reactions but no higher risk of serious adverse events. This vaccine is recommended for persons aged 65 years or older.
  iii. Quadrivalent inactivated influenza vaccine, cell culture-based (ccIIV4)—contraindications and precautions are the same as those for IIV4. It is not licensed for use in children younger than 18 years of age.
  iv. Recombinant influenza vaccine (RIV)—this is the only influenza vaccine that is egg-free. It is contraindicated in anyone with a history of a severe allergic

reaction to any vaccine component, but it is safe for use in individuals with serious egg allergy. It is not licensed for use in children younger than 18 years of age.

v. Quadrivalent live, attenuated, cold adapted influenza vaccine (LAIV)—given as a nasal spray. This vaccine is recommended only for healthy persons 2 to 49 years of age. Contraindications include pregnancy, hives or anaphylaxis to egg or egg products, persons with known or suspected immunodeficiencies, and children aged 2 through 4 years who have asthma or who have had a wheezing episode noted in the medical record within the past 12 months or for whom parents report that a health care provider stated that they had wheezing or asthma within the past 12 months.

Egg-Allergic Patients

Egg allergy of any severity (including anaphylaxis) is no longer considered a contraindication or precaution to receiving any injectable inactivated (IIV) or live, attenuated, intranasal (LAIV) influenza vaccines. Multiple published studies involving more than 4,100 egg-allergic patients (including those with severe anaphylactic reactions to egg) who have received IIV and more than 1,200 egg-allergic patients who have received LAIV have shown that these patients have tolerated the vaccines well with no hives or anaphylaxis. The CDC and the AAP Committee on Infectious Diseases have reviewed the data and believe that the data support that egg allergy does not impart an increased risk of anaphylactic reaction to immunization with either IIV or LAIV. Immediate hypersensitivity reactions such as urticarial or anaphylaxis may occur; however, the rates are no more common in egg-allergic than non-egg-allergic vaccine recipients. Anaphylactic reactions after influenza vaccine occur at the same rate as with other vaccines (approximately 1 per 1 million persons vaccinated) whether the recipient is egg allergic or not and whether the vaccine contains egg or not. Special precautions regarding the medical setting and waiting period after administration of IIV or LAIV to egg-allergic recipients beyond those recommended for any vaccine are not warranted. Persons with egg allergy of any severity can be safely vaccinated with IIV or LAIV in any setting.

Efficacy

The efficacy and effectiveness of influenza vaccines depend primarily on the age and immunocompetence of the vaccine recipients and the degree of similarity between the viruses in the vaccine and those circulating in the community. Efficacy in persons 2 years of age or older typically ranges from 50% to 80%.

Duration of Protection

Duration of protection 6 to 12 months—annual vaccination is critical to maintain protection against influenza in all populations.

Contraindications and Precautions to Influenza Vaccines

Contraindications
1. For inactivated, recombinant, and live, attenuated vaccines
    a. Severe allergic reaction (e.g., anaphylaxis) after previous dose of any influenza vaccine; or to a vaccine component

2. Additional contraindications for live, attenuated vaccine
    a. Pregnant women
    b. Immunocompromised persons, including but not limited to medications, congenital or acquired immunodeficiency states, HIV infection, anatomic or functional asplenia
    c. Close contacts and caregivers of severely immunosuppressed persons who require a protected environment
    d. Persons who have taken influenza antiviral medications (within the previous 48 hours for oseltamivir and zanamivir, 5 days for peramivir, and 17 days for baloxavir); avoid use of these antiviral drugs for 14 days after vaccination
    e. Asthma or a wheezing episode noted in the medical record within the past 12 months in children 2 through 4 years of age

Precautions
1. For inactivated, recombinant, and live, attenuated vaccines
    a. Moderate or severe acute illness with or without fever
    b. History of Guillain–Barré syndrome within 6 weeks of previous influenza vaccination
2. Additional precautions for live, attenuated vaccine
    a. Asthma in persons aged 5 years or older
    b. Other chronic medical conditions, such as other chronic lung disease, chronic cardiovascular disease (excluding isolated hypertension), diabetes, chronic renal or hepatic disease, hematologic disease, neurologic disease, and metabolic disorders

Frequently Asked Questions

What are the benefits of the flu vaccine?
Flu vaccination reduces the risk of influenza illness in recipients and protects those around recipients who may be more vulnerable to serious flu illness. Influenza vaccination also may make illness milder if someone does get sick and reduce the risk of more serious outcomes, such as hospitalizations and deaths. Studies have shown that flu vaccine reduced children's risk of flu-related pediatric intensive care unit admission by 74% and flu-related hospitalizations among adults by 71% during the 2011–2012 flu season. Vaccination has been associated with lower rates of some cardiac events among people with heart disease, especially among those who had had a cardiac event in the past year.

Does protection from seasonal influenza vaccine decline several months after vaccination? Should I wait until flu season starts to vaccinate my elderly or medically frail patients?
Antibody to seasonal inactivated influenza vaccine does decline in the months following vaccination, but it should still be high enough to provide protection through the end of the season. Because the onset of flu season is unpredictable, seasonal influenza vaccine should be administered ideally by October. To avoid missed opportunities, offer vaccination during routine health care visits and hospitalizations when vaccine is available.

How long does immunity from seasonal influenza vaccine last?
Protection from influenza vaccine usually persists for about a year, although antibody persistence may be shorter for persons aged 65 years or older. Vaccination is recommended on an

annual basis because of waning antibody titers and because of changes in the circulating influenza viruses from year to year.

When should I stop offering influenza vaccination?
Continue to offer flu vaccine as long as influenza viruses are circulating in the community. The peak of influenza activity usually occurs in January or February in the United States. It is recommended that providers continue to vaccinate persons into the spring (typically through May).

If an unvaccinated patient has just recovered from a confirmed case of influenza, should that person be vaccinated with influenza vaccine?
Yes. Influenza vaccines contain three or four influenza strains—two influenza A strains and one or two influenza B strains. Infection with one virus type does not confer immunity to other virus types, and it is not unusual to be exposed to more than one strain during a typical influenza season. So a person who recently had influenza will benefit from a vaccine containing additional influenza virus strains.

Is Guillain-Barré syndrome (GBS) an important risk for patients receiving influenza vaccination?
A significantly increased risk of GBS was reported in association with the swine flu vaccine in 1976. The reasons for that are unclear, but since that time, the risk of GBS following flu vaccination has been estimated to be approximately 1 in 1 million flu vaccine recipients. GBS is a risk following stimulation of the immune system whether by immunization or illness. Influenza illness is associated with a significantly greater risk of GBS than influenza vaccination, and the overall benefits of influenza vaccination far outweigh the risk of GBS.

Is influenza vaccine safe to administer to patients with multiple sclerosis?

Yes. Multiple sclerosis is not a contraindication to receiving any vaccine, including influenza vaccine. These patients should receive the inactivated influenza vaccine and not the live, attenuated influenza vaccine.

What type of influenza vaccine is recommended for pregnant women?

Pregnant women can receive any of the inactivated injectable vaccines. They should not be given the live, attenuated intranasal influenza vaccine. It is important to vaccinate pregnant women during any trimester because of the increased risk of influenza-related complications, hospitalizations, and death. Vaccinating pregnant women protects the woman, her unborn baby, and the baby following birth from influenza disease.

What vaccine, if any, should I offer a patient with a history of egg allergy?

Any flu vaccine (egg-based or non-egg-based) that is otherwise appropriate for the recipient's age and health status can be used. Egg allergy does not indicate additional safety measures for flu vaccination beyond those recommended for any recipient of any vaccine, regardless of severity of previous reaction to egg.

What is the value of high-dose flu vaccine?

High-dose flu vaccine has been associated with significantly higher antibody responses and better protection against laboratory-confirmed influenza illness (preventing an additional 24% laboratory-confirmed influenza illness in one large study) in persons aged 65 years or older.

What influenza vaccine should elderly individuals aged 65 years or older receive?
The CDC has made a preferential recommendation that elderly individuals aged 65 years or older receive high-dose, recombinant, or adjuvanted influenza vaccine.

Who should not receive the live, attenuated influenza vaccine?
The following persons should not receive LAIV:

- Children younger than age 2 years
- Adults aged 50 years or older
- Children aged 2 through 4 years with a wheezing episode during the preceding 12 months
- Persons with asthma
- Children and adults who have chronic pulmonary, cardiovascular (except isolated hypertension), renal, hepatic, neurologic/neuromuscular, hematologic, or metabolic disorders
- Immunosuppressed children and adults (including immunosuppression caused by medications or by HIV)
- Pregnant women

Patients will refuse influenza vaccination because they insist they "got the flu" after receiving the injectable vaccine in the past. How can I respond?
This misconception persists for several reasons. First, less than 1% of persons vaccinated with the injectable inactivated influenza vaccine develop flulike symptoms, such as mild fever and muscle aches, after vaccination. These side effects are not the same as having influenza infection, but people commonly confuse the symptoms as being the same.

Second, protective immunity does not develop until 1 or 2 weeks after vaccination. Some people vaccinated later in the season may be infected with influenza virus shortly after receiving the vaccine before immunity is established. Third, many people believe that "the flu" is any illness with fever and cold symptoms. If they get any viral respiratory illness, they blame it on the vaccine or believe that got "the flu" despite being vaccinated. Influenza vaccine protects against certain influenza viruses, not all viruses. Fourth, the influenza vaccine is not 100% effective, especially in older adults.

Can high-dose influenza vaccine be administered to patients younger than 65 years of age with chronic underlying conditions (e.g., HIV, immunodeficiency)?
No. The high-dose influenza vaccine is only licensed for persons aged 65 years or older and is not recommended for younger persons with underlying medical conditions.

Can a person aged 65 years or older who has already received a standard-dose influenza vaccine also receive a dose of high-dose influenza vaccine in the same influenza season?
No. It is not recommended that anyone receive more than one dose of influenza vaccine in the same season except for infants and children aged 6 months to 8 years who are receiving influenza vaccine for the first time and for whom 2 doses of vaccine are recommended.

How soon after a bone marrow transplant can patients be vaccinated against influenza?
Inactivated influenza vaccine should be administered beginning 6 months after bone marrow transplant and annually thereafter.

Which health care providers should be vaccinated against influenza?
It is important to vaccinate *all* hospital, outpatient, nursing home, and chronic care facility health care personnel with influenza vaccine, especially those who have direct patient contact. Vaccine response is diminished in elderly and immunosuppressed persons, and evidence suggests vaccinating health care personnel may be even more effective in preventing disease in hospital, nursing home, and chronic care facility residents than vaccinating the patients themselves.

Which health care personnel can receive the live, attenuated influenza vaccine (LAIV)?
LAIV can be administered to all health care personnel for whom it is indicated based on age and health history except those who care for severely immunocompromised patients in a protected (reverse airflow) environment.

If a patient is allergic to chicken or duck feathers, is this a contraindication to receiving an egg-based influenza vaccine?
No.

Can LAIV be administered to persons with a mild upper respiratory infection with or without fever?
Yes, unless it is clinically deemed that the patient's nasal congestion would interfere with the delivery of the vaccine to the nasopharyngeal mucosa. In this case, administration of the vaccine should be deferred until the congestion resolves.

Can a woman who is breastfeeding receive LAIV?

Yes. Breastfeeding is not a contraindication for the receipt of any routine vaccine, including LAIV. Postpartum maternal vaccination against influenza is associated with a significant reduction in illness, doctor visits, and antibiotic prescriptions in infants during influenza season.

Can LAIV be given to contacts of immunosuppressed patients?

Household members, health care personnel, and others with close contact to severely immunosuppressed individuals during periods in which the immunosuppressed person requires care in a protective environment should preferentially receive inactivated influenza vaccine.

What should be done in the situation in which a young patient is only able to receive half the dose of LAIV?

A half dose of LAIV or any vaccine is a nonstandard dose and should not be counted. If the second half of the dose is not administered at the same appointment, another full dose of influenza vaccine should be administered at another time. A dose of inactivated influenza vaccine can be administered at any time after the half dose of LAIV. If LAIV is given again, wait 4 weeks before administering another live vaccine.

What should be done is the situation in which a patient believes they had a reaction to the influenza vaccine in the past and requests that the vaccine dose be split into 2 doses administered on different days?

This is not an acceptable practice. Doses of influenza vaccine or any other vaccine should not be split in half or partial doses. If a half or partial dose is administered, it is not counted as a valid dose and should be repeated as soon as possible with a full age-appropriate vaccine dose.

Which persons who are traveling abroad should be given influenza vaccine?
Health care providers should vaccinate any person who failed to get vaccinated during the influenza season and who wants to reduce their risk of acquiring influenza during their travels. This includes persons who are traveling to the tropics, traveling with organized tourist groups at any time of the year, or traveling in the Southern Hemisphere from April through September.

If a patient received a dose of influenza vaccine in May for international travel, how long should the patient wait before getting vaccinated with the next season's influenza vaccine?
There should be a minimum of 4 weeks between the doses of influenza vaccine.

If a child needs 2 doses of influenza vaccine, can they receive 1 dose of injectable vaccine and 1 dose of the nasal spray vaccine?
Yes, as long as the child is eligible to receive nasal spray vaccine, it is acceptable to receive 1 dose of each type of influenza vaccine as long as the doses are spaced at least 4 weeks apart.

If high-dose influenza vaccine is not available, can 2 doses of standard-dose influenza vaccine be given to a person aged 65 years or older in place of the high-dose influenza vaccine?
No. This is not the same as high-dose influenza vaccine and is not recommended.

REFERENCES

Centers for Disease Control and Prevention. Prevention and control of seasonal influenza with vaccines: Recommendations of the Advisory Committee on Immunization Practices (ACIP)—United States, 2024–25. *MMWR Recomm Rep.* 2024;73(No. RR-5):1–25.

Des Roches A, Paradis L, Gagmon R, et al. Egg-allergic patients can be safely vaccinated against influenza. *J Allergy Clin Immunol.* 2012;130:1213–1216.

Des Roches A, Samaan K, Graham F, et al. Safe vaccination of patients with egg allergy by using live attenuated influenza vaccine. *J Allergy Clin Immunol Pract.* 2015;3:138–139.

Greenhawt M, Turner PJ, Kelso JM. Administration of influenza vaccines to egg allergic recipients: A practice parameter update 2017. *Ann Allergy Asthma Immunol.* 2018;120(1):49–52.

Joint Task Force on Practice Parameters. Update on influenza vaccination of egg allergic patients. *Ann Allergy Asthma Immunol.* 2013;111:301–302.

Kelso JM. Administering influenza vaccine to egg-allergic persons. *Expert Rev Vaccines.* 2014;13:1049–1057.

Turner PJ, Southern J, Andrews NJ, et al. Safety of live, attenuated influenza vaccine in atopic children with egg allergy. *J Allergy Clin Immunol.* 2015;136:376–381.

Turner PJ, Southern J, Andrews NJ, et al. Safety of live, attenuated influenza vaccine in young people with egg allergy: Multicenter prospective cohort study. *BMJ.* 2015;351:h6291.

HEPATITIS A

Did you know that:

- In 1988, an epidemic of hepatitis A in Shanghai, China, attributed to the consumption of raw clams affected 300,000 persons in a 2-month period.
- Hepatitis A vaccination was first introduced in the United States in 1995, expanded to 17 "high-risk" states in 1999, and expanded to all children aged 12 to 23 months of age in 2006. Following years of significant decline, the incidence of

hepatitis A increased annually from 2015 to 2019. This was attributed to widespread outbreaks primarily due to person-to-person transmission among persons reporting drug use or homelessness. The incidence of hepatitis A decreased 43% from 2020 to 2021, but this decrease may have been related to fewer people seeking health care and being tested for viral hepatitis during the COVID-19 pandemic.

Hepatitis A virus is the cause of 20% to 40% of viral hepatitis cases in the Western world. The majority (>70%) of cases in infants and children younger than 6 years of age are asymptomatic. Hepatitis A is the cause of an acute, self-limited illness associated with fever, malaise, jaundice, anorexia, and nausea that resolves in 2 months or less. Ten percent to 15% of symptomatic persons have prolonged or relapsing disease that may last as long as 6 months.

Hepatitis A infection in pregnancy may be associated with a high risk of maternal complications, including premature contractions, preterm labor, premature rupture of membranes, placental separation, vaginal bleeding, fetal distress, and low-birth-weight infants.

The hepatitis A vaccine was introduced in 1995, and health professionals now routinely vaccinate all children, travelers to certain countries, and persons at risk for the disease. Most cases of hepatitis A in the United States result from person-to-person transmission during communitywide outbreaks. In 2018, approximately 12,500 cases of hepatitis A were reported to the CDC from throughout the United States, representing a substantial increase from 2017. Persons at risk for acquiring hepatitis A infection or having severe infection are international travelers, men who have sex with men, persons who use injection or noninjection drugs, persons who anticipate close personal contact with an international adoptee, persons experiencing homelessness, persons with HIV infection, persons with chronic liver disease, persons living in group settings for those with developmental disabilities, and persons who are incarcerated.

Transmission

1. Direct person-to-person contact via fecal–oral route
2. Ingestion of contaminated food or water
3. Oral or anal sex

Hepatitis A viruses persist in the environment and can withstand food-production processes routinely used to inactivate bacterial pathogens.

Incubation Period

Incubation period is on average 28 days (range: 15–50 days).

Prevention

Post-exposure
   a. Administration of intramuscular immunoglobulin—if given within 2 weeks after exposure is greater than 85% effective in preventing symptomatic hepatitis A infection. Recommended to be administered to persons younger than 12 months of age, persons of any age who are immunocompromised or have chronic liver disease, and is preferred for persons 41 years of age or older.
   b. Hepatitis A vaccine—if given within 2 weeks after exposure is greater than 85% effective in preventing symptomatic hepatitis A infection. Recommended to be administered to

persons 12 months through 40 years of age. May be used in persons 41 years of age or older if immunoglobulin not available.

Pre-exposure
    a. Hepatitis A vaccine—licensed for persons 12 months of age or older.
    b. Hepatitis A vaccine may be given to infants between 6 and 12 months of age who are traveling abroad. This dose does not count toward the 2-dose recommended series.
    c. Immunoglobulin—persons younger than 6 months of age.

Vaccine: Given intramuscularly as a 2-dose series at 0 and 12 to 18 months of age. Vaccine should not be given to persons with hypersensitivity to any of the vaccine components.

Immunogenicity

95% after 1 dose; >99% after 2 doses

Duration of Protection

At least 20 years after 2-dose series, but probably lifelong. No additional booster doses beyond the 2-dose primary immunization series are recommended.

Contraindications and Precautions to Hepatitis A Vaccine

Contraindications
Severe allergic reaction (e.g., anaphylaxis) after a previous dose or to a vaccine component.

Precautions
Moderate or severe acute illness with or without fever.

Frequently Asked Questions

How stable is hepatitis A virus (HAV) in the environment?
Depending on the environmental conditions, HAV can remain stable in the environment for months. Heating foods at temperatures greater than 185°F (85°C) for 1 minute or disinfecting surfaces with a 1:100 dilution of bleach in tap water will inactivate HAV.

Can people with HAV develop chronic disease?
Unlike hepatitis B and hepatitis C viruses, HAV does not cause chronic, long-term infection. Once you have had HAV infection and recover, you cannot get it again.

Should prevaccination testing be performed before administering hepatitis A vaccine?
Prevaccination testing is recommended only in specific circumstances to reduce the costs of vaccinating people who are already immune to hepatitis A, including adults who were either born in or lived for extensive periods in geographic areas with high or intermediate hepatitis A endemicity. Hepatitis A vaccination should not be postponed if vaccination history is unavailable or if prevaccination testing is not possible. Vaccinating persons immune from natural infection carries no known risk, nor does giving extra doses of hepatitis A vaccine.

Should post-vaccination HAV titers be performed after a person has received the 2-dose vaccine series?

No. Post-vaccination testing is *not* indicated because of the high rate of vaccine response among vaccine recipients. Also, not all testing methods approved for diagnostic use in the United States have the sensitivity to detect low, but protective, anti-HAV concentrations after vaccination.

Should health care workers (HCWs) be routinely vaccinated against hepatitis A?

No. Studies have shown that HCWs are not at increased risk of HAV infection due to their occupation. The only HCWs for whom hepatitis A vaccine is routinely recommended are those who work with live HAV or with primates.

Should day care workers be routinely vaccinated against hepatitis A?

No. Childcare centers may be the source of outbreaks of hepatitis A in certain communities, but HAV disease in child care centers more commonly reflects transmission from the community.

Can a breastfeeding woman receive hepatitis A vaccine?

Yes. Hepatitis A vaccine is an inactivated vaccine that poses no harm to the breastfeeding infant.

What should be done in the situation in which an adult patient inadvertently receives a dose of pediatric hepatitis A vaccine?

As a general rule, if a patient is given a vaccine dose that is less than a full age-appropriate dose of any vaccine, the dose is invalid and the patient should be revaccinated with the age-appropriate dose as soon as feasible. However, there are two exceptions to the general rule:

1. If a patient sneezes after receiving nasal spray live, attenuated influenza vaccine, the dose is counted as valid.
2. If an infant regurgitates, spits up, or vomits during or after receiving oral rotavirus vaccine, the dose is counted as valid.

If a patient receives more than an age-appropriate dose of a vaccine (e.g., infant receiving adult dose of HAV), the dose is counted as valid and caution must be taken not to repeat the error. Using larger than recommended doses can be hazardous because of excessive local or systemic concentrations of antigens or other vaccine constituents.

Can someone donate blood if they have had hepatitis A?
If a patient had hepatitis A, they can donate blood when fully recovered—typically 6 to 12 months after recovery or documented HAV RNA negative and HAV IgG positive after recovery.

When does protection from hepatitis A vaccine commence?
Protection begins approximately 2 to 4 weeks after the first vaccine dose. A second booster dose results in long-term protection.

Your patient is leaving for their trip abroad in a few days. Can they still get the hepatitis A vaccine?

The first dose of hepatitis A vaccine can be given at any time before departure and will provide some protection for most healthy people.

Who should receive post-exposure prophylaxis (PEP) after exposure to hepatitis A?
People who might benefit from PEP include those who

- live with someone who has hepatitis A;
- have recently had sexual contact with someone who has hepatitis A;
- have recently shared injection or non-injection illegal drugs with someone who has hepatitis A;
- have had ongoing, close personal contact with a person with hepatitis A, such as a regular babysitter or caregiver; or
- have been exposed to food or water known to be contaminated with HAV.

Is it harmful to administer an extra dose(s) of hepatitis A vaccine or to repeat the entire vaccine series if documentation of vaccination history is unavailable?
No. If necessary, administering extra doses of hepatitis A vaccine is not harmful.

What are the current CDC guidelines for post-exposure protection against hepatitis A?
Persons who have recently been exposed to HAV and who have not been vaccinated previously should be administered a single dose of hepatitis A vaccine or immune globulin (IG; 0.02 mL/kg) as soon as possible and within 2 weeks after exposure.

- For healthy persons aged 12 months to 40 years, hepatitis A vaccine is preferred to IG because of the vaccine's advantages (long-term protection, ease of administration, and equivalent efficacy).
- For persons aged 40 years or older, IG is preferred because of the absence of data regarding vaccine performance in this age group and because of the more severe manifestations of hepatitis A in older adults.
- Vaccine can be used if IG cannot be obtained.
- IG should be used for children aged younger than 12 months, immunocompromised persons, persons with chronic liver disease, and persons who are allergic to the vaccine.

HEPATITIS B

Did you know that:

- Despite the availability of an effective vaccine, worldwide, hepatitis B virus (HBV) infection kills a person every 30 to 45 seconds.
- HBV is 100 times more infectious than HIV.
- An estimated 300 million people worldwide are chronically infected with HBV, and 15% to 40% will develop severe serious sequelae (e.g., cirrhosis, liver failure, and hepatocellular carcinoma) during their lifetime.

There are an estimated 46,000 new cases of HBV infection reported each year in the United States; however, the CDC recognizes that this only accounts for 10% of the cases. Adults 30 to 49 years of age account for the majority of the new cases being reported. Hepatitis B infection accounts for 2,000 to 4,000 deaths each year, primarily due to cirrhosis and liver cancer. The likelihood of developing symptoms of acute hepatitis is age-dependent: <1% of infants younger than 1 year of age, 5% to 15% of children 1 to 5 years of age, and 30% to 50% of people older than 5 years of age are symptomatic. The spectrum of signs and symptoms includes subacute illness with nonspecific symptoms (e.g., anorexia, nausea, or malaise); clinical hepatitis with jaundice or fulminant hepatitis; and extrahepatic manifestations such as arthralgia, arthritis, macular rashes, thrombocytopenia, polyarteritis nodosa, glomerulonephritis, or papular acrodermatitis (Gianotti–Crosti syndrome).

Risk factors for hepatitis B infection include the following:

- Travelers to countries where HBV infection is highly endemic
- Persons adopting or fostering children from countries where HBV infection is highly endemic
- Household contacts and sexual partners of person with HBV acute infection or chronic carriers
- Tattooing, piercing, or other forms of body modification
- Health care and public safety workers exposed to blood and other fluids
- Staff and patients of institutions for the developmentally disabled, assisted-living facilities, and nursing homes
- Correctional facilities
- Persons with end-stage renal disease, chronic liver disease, diabetes mellitus, HIV, or hemodialysis patients
- Men who have sex with men
- Persons seeking evaluation or treatment for a sexually transmitted infection, especially HIV and syphilis

- Current or recent injection-drug users
- Sexually active persons with multiple sexual partners

60% of persons infected with HBV *do not* have an identifiable risk factor.

Age at time of acute infection is the primary determinant of the risk of progression to chronic infection:

- Risk is 5% if HBV infection is acquired as an adult.
- Risk is 30% to 50% if the infection is acquired as a child younger than 5 years of age.
- Risk is >90% if infection is acquired as a neonate.

Transmission

Hepatitis B is transmitted through percutaneous and permucosal exposure to infected blood and body fluids (including serum, semen, vaginal secretions, cerebrospinal fluid, and synovial, pleural, pericardial, peritoneal, and amniotic fluids), with serum, semen, vaginal secretions, and amniotic fluid being the most infectious. The most common modes of transmission are parenteral, sexual, and perinatal.

Incubation Period

Incubation period is on average 90 days (range: 45–160 days). Women who are pregnant and have an acute hepatitis B infection are at increased risk for having a premature or low-birth-weight infant. Universal screening of *all* pregnant women for hepatitis B surface antigen (HbsAg), regardless of HBV vaccination history, is strongly recommended and should be performed during an early prenatal visit with every pregnancy.

Perinatal transmission poses an extremely high risk to the infant for developing chronic disease and its complications. There are an estimated 20,000 infants each year born to women known to be infected with HBV infection (remember that only 10% of cases in adults are reported, so the vast majority of cases are unrecognized). Perinatal transmission of HBV is highly efficient and usually occurs from blood exposure during labor and delivery. In the absence of post-exposure treatment, 6,000 of the 20,000 infants would develop chronic infection, and 25% will die prematurely from HBV-related hepatocellular carcinoma or cirrhosis.

If a mother is HbsAg-positive at time of delivery, 20% of infants born to these mothers will be infected with HBV—in the absence of post-exposure treatment, 90% of these infants will go on to become chronic carriers.

If a mother is HbsAg-positive *and* HbeAg-positive (marker for transmissibility—very high viral loads) at the time of delivery, 70% to 90% of infants born to these mothers will be infected with HBV—in the absence of post-exposure treatment, >90% of these infants will go on to become chronic carriers.

Prevention

Post-exposure

a. Perinatal—hepatitis B immune globulin (HBIG) given within 12 hours of birth *and* dose of HBV vaccine—use of this regimen is 95% effective in preventing transmission of HBV to infant. Standard immune globulin is *not* effective for post-exposure prophylaxis against HBV infection because concentrations of hepatitis B antibodies are too low.

b. Discrete exposure to an HBsAg-positive source (e.g., percutaneous—needlestick, bite, non-intact skin or

mucosal exposure to HbsAg-positive blood or body fluids; sexual contact or needle sharing with HbsAg-positive person; victim of sexual assault/abuse by a person who is HbsAg-positive)—HBIG and hepatitis B vaccine to complete series.
c. Household contact of HbsAg-positive person or exposure to a source with unknown HBsAg status—administer hepatitis B vaccine series.

Pre-exposure
a. Administer hepatitis B vaccine series (Engerix B and Recombivax HB)—given intramuscularly as 3-dose series at 0-, 1-, and 6-month intervals.
b. Administer hepatitis B vaccine series (Heplislav-B)—given intramuscularly as 2-dose series at 0- and 1-month intervals. Only approved for use in persons 18 years of age or older.
c. PreHevbrio (VBI Vaccines) is an HBsAg recombinant vaccine with aluminum hydroxide adjuvant that was approved by the U.S. Food and Drug Administration (FDA) in 2021 for use in people 18 years of age or older. It is given as a 3-dose series (1.0 mL dose at 0, 1, and 6 months) and administered intramuscularly.

Vaccine Efficacy

Efficacy is 90% to 95% after 2- or 3-dose series for preventing HBV infection and clinical HBV disease.

Duration of Protection

At least 20 years but probably lifelong. Confers protection against clinical illness and chronic HBV infection.

Contraindications and Precautions to Hepatitis B Vaccine

Contraindications
1. Severe allergic reaction (e.g., anaphylaxis) after a previous dose or to a vaccine component.

Precautions
1. Moderate or severe acute illness with or without fever.

Frequently Asked Questions

Can hepatitis B virus (HBV) be transmitted in the day care setting by the saliva of drooling infants?
HBV has been found in saliva, but there are no data indicating that saliva exposure alone can transmit an HBV infection. If an HBV-infected person bites another person, HBV can be transmitted; however, it is the blood in the infected person's mouth from the bite that was the likely vehicle of transmission. HBV is not spread by casual contact, sneezing, kissing, coughing, sharing eating utensils or drinking containers, or by food or water.

Can a patient who had an acute hepatitis B infection that was completely resolved ever get hepatitis B infection again?
In general, the answer is no. However, it is possible for this person to acquire a different HBV variant or subtype as the cause of the second infection. This would be a very rare occurrence.

I run a clinic for patients who are chronic hepatitis B carriers. How stable is HBV in the environment, and what type

of disinfectant should I use to clean my waiting room and exam rooms?
HBV is very stable in the environment and remains viable for 7 or more days on environmental surfaces at room temperature. It is capable of transmitting HBV infection despite the absence of visible blood. Any disinfectant that is tuberculocidal will kill HBV.

What screening blood test should be done in pregnant women to prevent perinatal HBV infection?
Screening should be done with the hepatitis B surface antigen (HBsAg) test only. This test will determine whether a woman currently has an HBV infection that she can transmit to her infant. Other HBV tests, such as antibody to hepatitis B core antigen (anti-HBc) and hepatitis B surface antibody (anti-HBs), are not useful when screening to prevent perinatal HBV infections and should not be used in the screening process.

Does a woman who has been previously vaccinated against HBV infection still need to screened for HBV during pregnancy?
Yes. Women who have received hepatitis B vaccine should still be screened for HBsAg early in each pregnancy. Just because she is vaccinated does not mean that she is HbsAg-negative.

Can a pregnant woman receive hepatitis B vaccine?
Yes. Current hepatitis B vaccines contain noninfectious HBsAg and pose no risk to the developing fetus.

How should an infant be managed if their mother's HBsAg test result is not available at the time of birth?

1. Women without documentation of HbsAg test results at the time of admission for delivery should have blood drawn and tested as soon as possible after admission.
2. All infants born to women without documentation of HbsAg test results should receive the first dose of single-antigen hepatitis B vaccine (without HBIG) by 12 hours of age.
3. If the mother is found to be HbsAg-positive, her infant should receive HBIG as soon as possible but no later than 7 days of age, and the HBV vaccine series should be completed according to the recommended schedule for infants born to HbsAg-positive mothers.
4. If the mother is found to be HbsAg-negative, the infant's HBV vaccine series should be completed according to the recommended schedule.

Is it safe for an HbsAg-positive mother to breastfeed her infant?
Yes. An HbsAg-positive mother should be encouraged to breastfeed her infant if she wishes to do so. The infant should receive HBIG and hepatitis B vaccine within 12 hours of birth. Even though HBV can be detected in breast milk, studies have shown that breastfed infants born to HbsAg-positive mothers do not have an increased rate of perinatal or early childhood HBV infection.

What should be done in the situation in which an infant inadvertently receives a dose of the adult formulation of hepatitis B vaccine?
The adult formation of hepatitis B vaccine contains twice the amount of antigen compared to a dose of the infant/child formulation. If an infant receives an adult dose of the hepatitis B vaccine, the dose is counted as valid and does not need to

be repeated. Hepatitis B vaccine is a very safe vaccine and no adverse events would be expected. The next age-appropriate dose should be given on the routine schedule.

Is post-vaccination serologic testing recommended for adults who receive hepatitis B vaccine?
Testing is not necessary after routine vaccination of adults. Serologic testing for immunity after vaccination is recommended only for people whose subsequent clinical management depends on knowledge of their immune status. Post-vaccination testing is recommended for health care and public safety workers at increased risk for continued exposure to blood on the job, immune compromised individuals, and sex and needle-sharing partners of HbsAg-positive persons. Testing should be performed 1 or 2 months after the last dose of vaccine. However, the CDC does not recommend routine testing of health care personnel who were not tested within the 1- or 2-month post-vaccination period. Health care personnel who are exposed to HBV can be tested as part of post-exposure management.

What should be done in the situation in which a person has received an appropriate 3-dose series of HBV vaccine but their anti-HBs (HBsAb) titer is negative (<10 mIU/mL)?
Give 1 dose of hepatitis B vaccine, and the person should be tested for anti-HBs 1 or 2 months after the dose of the vaccine. If the anti-HBs test is still negative after dose of vaccine, the person should be tested for HBsAg and anti-HBc to determine their HBV infection status. People who test negative for HBsAg and anti-HBc should be considered vaccine non-responders and susceptible to HBV infection. These patients should be counseled about precautions to prevent HBV infection and the need to obtain HBIG prophylaxis for any known

or likely exposure to HBsAg-positive blood. Persons found to be HbsAg-negative but anti-HBc-positive were infected in the past and require no vaccination or treatment.

Can a different brand be used to complete a vaccination series started with Engerix-B or Recombivax HB?
A hepatitis B vaccine series that was begun with one brand of hepatitis B vaccine may be completed with a different brand. When feasible, the same manufacturer's vaccines should be used to complete the series. However, vaccination should not be deferred when the manufacturer of the previously administered vaccine is unknown or when the vaccine from the same manufacturer is unavailable.

MEASLES

Did you know that:

- The 7-year-old daughter of Roald Dahl, the British author of *Charlie and the Chocolate Factory*, died from a measles infection in 1962, the year before a measles vaccine became available. Dahl went on to become a strong supporter of vaccines: "In my opinion parents who now refuse to have their children immunized are putting the lives of those children at risk. In America, where measles immunization is compulsory, measles like smallpox, has been virtually wiped out. Here in Britain, because so many parents refuse, either out of obstinacy or ignorance or fear, to allow their children to be immunized, we still have a hundred thousand cases of measles every year."

- Currently on a worldwide basis, 13 people die from measles every hour; measles continues to kill 430 children each day.
- One person with measles can transmit the illness to up to 18 susceptible other individuals, making it the most infectious vaccine-preventable disease.

Measles virus causes an acute viral illness characterized by fever, cough, conjunctivitis, coryza, pharyngitis, erythematous maculopapular rash (starts on forehead around hairline and spreads centrifugally from the head to the feet, becoming confluent), lymphadenopathy (cervical, suboccipital, and postauricular), and Koplik spots (white lesions on an erythematous base on buccal mucosa opposite the upper molars). It is one of the most contagious viral infections, with secondary attack rates of greater than 90% in susceptible household contacts.

Complications

Complications include otitis media; diarrhea; bronchopneumonia (responsible for 60% of deaths associated with measles disease and may be measles virus associated and/or a secondary bacterial superinfection with *Streptococcus pneumoniae*, Group A streptococcus, and *Staphylococcus aureus*); acute encephalitis (more common in adults, associated with fever, headache, seizures, altered consciousness, permanent neurologic sequelae, and brain damage); and subacute sclerosing panencephalitis (SSPE). SSPE is a rare degenerative central nervous disease that generally occurs 7 to 10 years after wild-type measles infection, especially in those who had measles before 2 years of age. It is caused by a persistent infection with a mutant measles-related virus in the central nervous system. It is characterized by behavioral and intellectual deterioration and seizures. In the vast majority of cases, it results in death 1 to 3 years after symptom onset.

Measles infection during pregnancy may be associated with a risk of miscarriage and prematurity. Pneumonia (both measles virus associated and secondary bacterial superinfection) is a major complication in pregnant women with measles.

Significant declines in measles vaccination rates or lack of measles vaccination in various areas of the world have resulted in a major resurgence in endemic disease. Yemen and India have had the highest number of measles cases in the world. Many countries in Europe, Asia, Africa, and South America, in addition to New Zealand, are also experiencing large numbers of measles cases. The majority of the cases seen in the United States are brought in by infected persons from other countries or by unvaccinated persons who contract the disease while traveling to countries where measles is endemic.

Transmission

The disease is transmitted person-to-person by direct contact with droplets from infected respiratory secretions. Persons are contagious from 4 days before the rash to 4 days after appearance of the rash.

Incubation Period

8 to 12 days

Prevention

Post-exposure
  a. Administration of immunoglobulin can be given to prevent or modify measles in a susceptible person within 6 days of

exposure. It is indicated for susceptible household or other close contacts of persons with measles, particularly contacts younger than 6 months of age, pregnant women, and immunocompromised people, for whom the risk of complications is highest, or in those persons in whom measles vaccine is contraindicated.
   b. MMR (measles, mumps, rubella) vaccine, if given within 72 hours of measles exposure, will provide protection in some cases. It may be given to individuals 6 months of age or older.

Pre-exposure
   a. MMR vaccine—live, attenuated vaccine containing measles, mumps, and rubella viruses. Recommended for use in persons born in 1957 or later, with first dose given to those 12 months of age or older.
   b. Given subcutaneously as MMR vaccine as a 2-dose series with minimal interval of 28 days between doses. In infants, first dose is given at 12 to 15 months of age, with second dose given at 4 to 6 years of age.
   c. Inadvertent administration of MMR vaccine to a pregnant woman is *not* an indication for termination of the pregnancy.
   d. May be administered to infants between 6 and 12 months of age who are traveling internationally or during outbreaks. This dose does not count toward the required 2-dose series.

Immunogenicity

95% after 1 dose; >99% after 2 doses

Duration of Protection

Lifelong after 2 doses

Contraindications and Precautions to MMR Vaccine

Contraindications
1. History of severe (anaphylactic) reaction to neomycin (or other vaccine component) or following a previous dose of MMR
2. Pregnancy
3. Severe immunosuppression from either disease or therapy

Precautions
1. Receipt of an antibody-containing blood product in the previous 11 months
2. Moderate or severe acute illness with or without fever
3. History of thrombocytopenia or thrombocytopenia purpura

Frequently Asked Questions

Why does being born before 1957 confer immunity to measles?
People born before 1957 lived through a number of years of epidemic measles before the first measles vaccine was licensed in 1963. Because of this, these people are very likely to have had measles disease. Data from survey studies suggest that 95% to 98% of those born before 1957 are immune to measles. However, if serologic testing indicates that the person is not immune, at least 1 dose of MMR should be administered.

What are the current CDC criteria for evidence of immunity to measles, mumps, and rubella?

The current CDC criteria for evidence of immunity to measles, mumps, and rubella are as follows:

1. Documented receipt of two appropriately timed doses of MMR vaccine, the first dose of which was given after 1 year of age
2. Laboratory confirmation of disease
3. Born before 1957

Physician diagnosis of disease has been removed as reliable evidence of immunity.

What should be done in the situation in which the MMR vaccine was given intramuscularly (IM) instead of subcutaneously (SC)?

It is recommended that all live injected vaccines (e.g., MMR, varicella, and yellow fever) be given SC; however, IM administration of these vaccines does not decrease immunogenicity, and doses given IM do *not* need to be repeated.

What should be done in the situation in which measles, mumps, rubella, and varicella (MMRV) vaccine was mistakenly given to an adult instead of MMR?

MMRV vaccine is licensed for use in persons 1 year to 12 years of age. If it is given to a patient 13 years of age or older, it is considered to be off-label use. This dose may be counted as valid toward the completion of the MMR and varicella vaccine series and does not need to be repeated.

What are the current CDC recommendations for the administration of a dose of MMR vaccine to infants 6 to 11 months of age who will be traveling internationally?
The CDC recommends that children who will be traveling or living abroad should be vaccinated with MMR vaccine at an earlier age than that recommended for children who live in the United States given that the risk for measles exposure can be high in both developed and developing countries. It is recommended that children aged 6 to 11 months receive 1 dose of MMR vaccine before departure from the United States. This dose does not count toward the 2 recommended doses of MMR at ages 12 to 15 months and 4 to 6 years.

Can MMR vaccine be given to a child whose sibling is receiving chemotherapy?
Yes. MMR and varicella vaccines should be given to the healthy household contacts of immunosuppressed patients.

Is egg allergy considered a contraindication to receiving MMR vaccine?
No. Studies have documented the safety of giving MMR vaccine (which is grown in chick embryo tissue culture) to children with severe egg allergy. Egg allergy is *not* considered a contraindication to MMR vaccine, and the CDC and AAP recommend routine MMR vaccination of egg-allergic children without the use of special protocols or desensitization procedures.

Can MMR vaccine be given to a breastfeeding mother or to a breastfed infant?
Yes, breastfeeding does not interfere with the response to MMR vaccine, and vaccination of a woman who is breastfeeding poses no risk to the infant being breastfed.

MUMPS

Did you know that:

- The clinical picture of mumps (*swelling about one or both ears and, in some instances, painful swelling of one or both testes*) was first described by Hippocrates in the 5th century BC in Book 1 of his *Book of Epidemics*.
- Orchitis, an inflammation of the testicles, occurs in approximately 25% of males who are infected with mumps after puberty. Up to 50% will develop testicular atrophy or shrinkage, and 10% will have a drop in their sperm count.

Mumps is a systemic disease usually characterized by swelling of one or more of the salivary glands, most commonly the parotid glands. Approximately one-third of the infections do not have clinically apparent salivary gland swelling and may be asymptomatic or manifest primarily as a respiratory tract infection. Infection in adults is much more likely to result in complications.

Complications

More than 50% of people with mumps have cerebrospinal fluid pleocytosis, but less than 10% have symptoms of viral meningitis. Symptoms are most commonly seen in older children, adolescents, and adults. Epididymo-orchitis is a complication reported in 30% to 38% of post-pubertal males, especially in the second, third, and fourth decades of life. It is usually unilateral but may be bilateral in up to 38% of cases. Oophoritis occurs in 7% of post-pubertal females. The incidence of deafness as a complication is 0.5 to 5 per 100,000 cases; it is usually unilateral and permanent.

Mumps infection during pregnancy is associated with increased rates of fetal mortality in women who contract mumps during the first trimester of pregnancy (27.3% vs. 13% in healthy controls). Although mumps virus can cross the placenta, this mortality is not associated with the development of fetal malformations. Other complications in pregnant women include mastitis, aseptic meningitis, and glomerulonephritis.

Large outbreaks have been seen in recent years on college campuses, among the Hasidic Jewish communities in New York and New Jersey, and among professional sports teams.

Transmission

Contact with infectious respiratory tract secretions and saliva. The period of maximum communicability is several days before and after the onset of parotid swelling.

Incubation Period

16 to 18 days

Prevention

Post-exposure
a. Immunoglobulin preparations are *not* effective as post-exposure prophylaxis for mumps.
b. MMR (measles, mumps, rubella) vaccine has *not* been demonstrated to be effective in preventing infection after exposure. MMR vaccine can be given after exposure because immunization will provide protection against subsequent exposures.

c. A third dose of MMR vaccine may be given during mumps outbreaks on college campuses as a measure to control the outbreak.

Pre-exposure

a. MMR vaccine—live, attenuated vaccine containing measles, mumps, and rubella viruses. Recommended for use in persons born in 1957 or later, with first dose given to those 12 months of age or older.

b. Given subcutaneously as MMR vaccine as a 2-dose series with minimal interval of 28 days between doses. In infants, first dose is given at 12 to 15 months of age, with second dose given at 4 to 6 years of age. Inadvertent administration of MMR vaccine to a pregnant woman is *not* an indication for termination of the pregnancy.

Immunogenicity

73% to 91% after 1 dose; 79% to 95% after 2 doses

Duration of Protection

Lifelong after 2 doses

Contraindications and Precautions to MMR Vaccine

Contraindications

1. History of severe (anaphylactic) reaction to neomycin (or other vaccine component) or following a previous dose of MMR
2. Pregnancy

3. Severe immunosuppression from either disease or therapy. This includes people with conditions such as congenital immunodeficiency, AIDS, leukemia, lymphoma, and generalized malignancy, and also those receiving treatment for cancer with drugs, radiation, or large doses of corticosteroids.

Precautions
1. Receipt of an antibody-containing blood product in the previous 11 months
2. Moderate or severe acute illness with or without fever
3. History of thrombocytopenia or thrombocytopenia purpura

Frequently Asked Questions

How long is a person with mumps contagious?
People with mumps are considered most infectious from a few days before until 5 days after the onset of parotitis (facial swelling). The CDC recommends isolating mumps patients for 5 days after their glands begin to swell.

Can someone who had a laboratory-confirmed case of mumps get mumps again?
People who have had mumps are usually protected for life against another mumps infection. However, second occurrences of mumps do rarely happen.

Which adult patients should receive 2 doses of MMR vaccine?
Certain adults are at higher risk of exposure to measles, mumps, and/or rubella and should receive a second dose of MMR unless they have other evidence of immunity; this includes adults who are

- students in postsecondary educational institutions;
- health care personnel;
- living in a community experiencing an outbreak or recently exposed to the disease; and
- planning to travel internationally (for measles and mumps).

People who received inactivated (killed) measles vaccine or measles vaccine of unknown type during the period 1963 to 1967 should be revaccinated with 2 doses of MMR vaccine. People vaccinated before 1979 with either killed mumps vaccine or mumps vaccine of unknown type who are at high risk for mumps infection (e.g., people who are working in a health care facility) should be considered for revaccination with 2 doses of MMR vaccine.

RUBELLA

Did you know that:

- Rubella, first described in the late 18th century as a mild exanthematous disease of children and young adults, exploded onto the world stage in 1941 when it was recognized as an important cause of congenital defects in the fetus after maternal infection during pregnancy.
- The sweat of patients with rubella smells like freshly plucked chicken feathers.

Rubella (German measles) is caused by rubella virus. The majority of postnatal rubella cases are subclinical and asymptomatic. Clinical disease is mild and characterized by a generalized erythematous maculopapular rash, lymphadenopathy, and low-grade fever. The rash starts on the face, becomes generalized over 24 hours, and lasts a median of 3 days. Lymphadenopathy, which may precede the rash, often involves the posterior auricular or suboccipital lymph nodes but can be generalized and lasts between 5 and 8 days. Transient polyarthralgia and polyarthritis are commonly seen in adolescents and adults, especially females. Due to the success of the vaccination program, the rubella cases seen in the United States occur in persons born in other countries who were never vaccinated or in underimmunized people.

Complications

Encephalitis (1 in 6,000 cases) and thrombocytopenia (1 in 3,000 cases). Rubella during pregnancy is associated with a higher incidence of miscarriage, fetal death, or the congenital rubella syndrome (a constellation of congenital anomalies). A pregnant woman infected with rubella in early pregnancy has up to a 90% chance of giving birth to a baby with congenital rubella syndrome. The most common clinical manifestations seen in the infant at the time of birth include "blueberry muffin" lesions, growth restriction, interstitial pneumonitis, hepatosplenomegaly, thrombocytopenia, and radiolucent bone lesions. The most common anomalies associated with the congenital rubella syndrome are ophthalmologic (cataracts, microphthalmia, congenital glaucoma), cardiac (patent ductus arteriosus, peripheral pulmonary artery stenosis), auditory (sensorineural hearing loss), and neurologic (meningoencephalitis, microcephaly, mental retardation).

Congenital defects occur in up to 85% of cases if maternal infection occurs during the first 12 weeks of gestation, 50% during the first 13 to 16 weeks of gestation, and 25% during the end of the second trimester.

Transmission

Direct or droplet contact from infected nasopharyngeal secretions. The period of maximal communicability occurs from a few days before to 7 days after the onset of rash.

Incubation Period

16 to 18 days

Prevention

Post-exposure
- a. Immunoglobulin preparations are *not* effective as post-exposure prophylaxis for rubella and are *not* recommended for routine post-exposure prophylaxis of rubella in early pregnancy or any other circumstance.
- b. MMR (measles, mumps, rubella) vaccine has *not* been demonstrated to be effective in preventing infection after exposure. MMR vaccine can be given after exposure because immunization will provide protection against subsequent exposures.

Post-exposure evaluation of the pregnant woman includes the following:

- a. Obtaining a blood sample as soon as possible after exposure and testing for rubella IgM and IgG antibodies. An aliquot of frozen serum should be stored for possible repeated testing at a later time. The presence of rubella-specific IgG antibody at the time of exposure indicates that the person is most likely immune.

b. If antibody is not detectable, a second blood specimen should be obtained 2 or 3 weeks later and tested concurrently with the first specimen.

c. If the second test result is negative, another blood specimen should be obtained 6 weeks after the exposure and also tested concurrently with the first specimen.

d. A **negative test result** in **both the second and third specimens** indicates that infection has *not* occurred.

e. A **positive test result** in the **second or third specimen** but *not* the **first** indicates a **recent** infection.

Pre-exposure
a. MMR vaccine—live, attenuated vaccine-containing measles, mumps, and rubella viruses. Recommended for use in persons born in 1957 or later, with first dose given to those 12 months of age or older. Contraindictated in persons who are pregnant, persons with certain immunodeficiencies, or those who had a previous anaphylactic reaction to the vaccine or any of its components.

Vaccine: Given subcutaneously as MMR vaccine as a 2-dose series with minimal interval of 28 days between doses. In infants, first dose is given at 12 to 15 months of age, with second dose given at 4 to 6 years of age. Inadvertent administration of MMR vaccine to a pregnant woman is *not* an indication for termination of the pregnancy.

Immunogenicity

73% to 91% after 1 dose; 79% to 95% after 2 doses

Duration of Protection

Lifelong after 2 doses

Contraindications and Precautions to MMR Vaccine

Contraindications
1. History of severe (anaphylactic) reaction to neomycin (or other vaccine component) or following a previous dose of MMR
2. Pregnancy
3. Severe immunosuppression from either disease or therapy

Precautions
1. Receipt of an antibody-containing blood product in the previous 11 months
2. Moderate or severe acute illness with or without fever
3. History of thrombocytopenia or thrombocytopenia purpura

Frequently Asked Questions

What is the recommended length of time a woman should wait after receiving MMR (rubella) vaccine before becoming pregnant?
The CDC recommends deferring pregnancy for 4 weeks after receiving MMR vaccine.

What should be done in the situation in which a pregnant woman inadvertently was given an MMR vaccine?
MMR vaccination during pregnancy alone is not a reason to terminate the pregnancy. No specific action needs to be taken other than to reassure the woman that no adverse outcomes are expected because of this vaccination.

What should be done in the situation in which a pregnant woman's rubella test result shows that she is "not immune"

but she has documentation of receiving 2 appropriately timed doses of MMR vaccine?
It is now recommended that women of childbearing age who have received 1 or 2 doses of a rubella-containing vaccine and have serum rubella IgG titers that are not positive should be administered 1 additional dose of MMR vaccine (maximum 3 doses) and do not need to be retested for serologic evidence of rubella immunity. MMR vaccine should not be administered to a pregnant woman. The dose should be given after the baby is delivered.

How soon after delivery can MMR vaccine be given?
MMR vaccine may be administered any time after delivery. It should be administered before hospital discharge, even if the patient has received RhoGam during the hospital stay, is discharged in less than 24 hours, or is breastfeeding.

Is there any evidence that MMR vaccine or thimerosal are causes of autism spectrum disorder (ASD)?
No. This is an issue that has been studied extensively, including several thorough reviews by the Institute of Medicine (IOM). A 2004 scientific review by IOM concluded that "the evidence favors rejection of a causal relationship between thimerosal-containing vaccines and ASD." Since 2003, there have been nine CDC-funded or conducted studies that have found no link between thimerosal-containing vaccines and ASD, as well as no link between the MMR vaccine and ASD in children. In 2011, an IOM report on eight routinely used vaccines (MMR, hepatitis A, meningococcal, varicella zoster, influenza, hepatitis B, HPV, and tetanus-containing vaccines) given to children and adults found that these vaccines are

very safe and that there is no link between receiving vaccines and developing ASD. A 2013 CDC study added to the research showing that vaccines do not cause ASD. The study examined the number of antigens (substances in vaccines that cause the body's immune system to produce disease-fighting antibodies) from vaccines during the first 2 years of life. The results showed that the total amount of antigen from vaccines received was the same between children with ASD and those who did not have ASD. All the extensive research performed to date shows absolutely no evidence of any link between receiving vaccines or those vaccines containing trace thimerosal and ASD.

How likely is it for a person to develop arthritis after receiving an MMR vaccine?
Joint pain or arthralgia and transient arthritis following MMR vaccination occur only in people who were susceptible to rubella at the time of vaccination. Approximately 25% of non-immune post-pubertal women report joint pain after receiving a rubella-containing vaccine, and approximately 10% to 30% report arthritis-like signs and symptoms. If joint symptoms occur, they generally do so 1 to 3 weeks after vaccination, are mild, and last approximately 2 days.

How soon must MMR vaccine be administered once it has been reconstituted with diluent?
Optimally, MMR vaccine should be administered immediately after reconstitution. If reconstituted, MMR vaccine should be used within 8 hours. If it is not used within this time period, it should be discarded. The dose should be refrigerated and should never be left at room temperature.

VARICELLA ZOSTER (CHICKENPOX)

Did you know that:

- In 2011, in a misguided attempt to expose their children to the chickenpox virus to build immunity later in life, a group of parents throughout the United States (Tennessee, Arizona, California) started trading chickenpox virus-laced lollipops by mail, which is illegal and a federal crime.
- Prior to the introduction of varicella vaccine, varicella accounted for 10,600 hospitalizations and 100 to 150 deaths each year in the United States. That equates to 1 or 2 deaths each week!
- Primary varicella infection (chickenpox) was not differentiated from smallpox until the end of the 18th century.
- Chickenpox vaccine became available in the United States in 1995. Yearly in the United States, more than 3.5 million cases, 9,000 hospitalizations, and 100 deaths are prevented by vaccination.

Primary infection with **varicella zoster virus (VZV)** results in varicella (chickenpox). VZV is a DNA virus and is a member of the herpesvirus family. Like other herpesviruses, VZV has the capacity to persist in the body after the primary infection. VZV establishes latency in the dorsal root ganglia after primary infection, and reactivation at a later time results in herpes zoster (shingles). Varicella is a highly contagious disease, with an 80% to 100% secondary household attack rate in unvaccinated persons. VSZ enters through the respiratory tract and conjunctiva. It replicates at the site of entry in the nasopharynx and regional lymph nodes. A primary viremia occurs 4 to 6 days after infection, and there is spread of the virus to other organs such as spleen, liver, and sensory ganglia. Further replication occurs in the viscera, followed by a secondary viremia with viral replication in the skin. The virus is believed to have a short survival in the environment.

Clinical Course

The appearance of the rash is preceded by a 1- or 2-day prodrome of fever, malaise, headache, and abdominal pain. The rash appears as crops of lesions that develop over several days. Each crop progresses within 24 hours from macules to papules to vesicles, then pustules before crusting. All lesions are on an erythematous base and are pruritic. Lesions are in different stages of development at any given time and classically are described as "dew drops on a rose petal." The rash usually starts on the face and trunk and then spreads to the extremities and all other areas of the body. Typically between 250 and 500 lesions develop and are usually crusted by 4 to 7 days after onset of the rash. Recovery from primary varicella usually results in lifetime immunity. Adults may have more severe disease and have a higher incidence of complications. Children with immunocompromising conditions may develop a severe progressive form of varicella characterized by high fever, extensive vesicular eruptions, high complication rates, and prolonged illness. In otherwise healthy persons, a second occurrence of varicella is uncommon, but it can happen if the person was younger than 6 months of age when they had the infection or the infection was very mild.

Complications include secondary bacterial infections of the skin lesions most commonly caused by group A streptococcus and *Staphylococcus aureus* (which may progress to necrotizing fasciitis); pneumonia (viral or bacterial), which occurs in 15% of adults and is the most common complication in this population; central nervous system manifestations (e.g., cerebellar ataxia, meningoencephalitis, encephalitis); hepatitis; thrombocytopenia; acute respiratory distress syndrome; and hemorrhagic complications.

Persons at the highest risk of complications of varicella include healthy adults, pregnant women, developing fetuses, infants born to mothers who have varicella 5 days before or after delivery, and immunocompromised persons of any age. The risk of varicella complications is 10 to 20 times higher in adults than in children.

Congenital varicella syndrome (fetal varicella syndrome) may occur in women, with maternal varicella infection occurring during the first two trimesters of pregnancy. There is an estimated 2% incidence of congenital disease after maternal varicella infection occurring in the first 20 weeks of gestation. Features of congenital varicella include low birth weight, skin lesions or scarring in a dermatomal distribution (76% of cases), neurologic defects such as microcephaly (60% of cases), ophthalmologic disease (51% of cases), skeletal anomalies (e.g., hypoplasia of the extremities), and muscle atrophy (50% of cases). Up to 30% of infants born with congenital varicella syndrome die in the first month of life (Table 11).

Transmission

Person to person by direct contact, inhalation of aerosols from vesicular fluid of skin lesions of acute varicella and/or zoster, or aerosolized respiratory tract secretions.

Incubation Period

Incubation period is 14 to 16 days after exposure to rash. The maximal period of contagiousness is 1 or 2 days before onset of the rash until all the lesions have crusted. In cases in which there

Table 11 TIMING OF MATERNAL VARICELLA INFECTION AND POTENTIAL OUTCOME IN FETUS

Period of Gestation of Infected Mother	Potential Outcome in the Fetus
7 to 28 weeks	Fetal varicella syndrome
1 to 28 weeks	Neonatal/childhood herpes zoster
2 weeks before delivery	Neonatal chickenpox
5 days before or after delivery[a]	Neonatal disseminated chickenpox with septicemia and increased mortality of up to 30%

[a]Potentially may be the most severe outcome for the fetus.

is only a maculopapular rash, the person is contagious until the rash disappears.

Prevention

Post-exposure

a. Varicella zoster immune globulin (VariZIG) administered intramuscularly from 4 to 10 days after exposure. Recommended dose is based on kilograms of body weight: 62.5 units (0.5 vial) for children weighing ≤2.0 kg; 125 units (1 vial) for children weighing 2.1 to 10 kg; 250 units (2 vials) for children weighing 10.1 to 20 kg; 375 units (3 vials) for children weighing 20.1 to 30 kg; 500 units (4 vials) for children weighing 30.1 to 40 kg; and 625 units (5 vials) for all people weighing >40 kg. If VariZIG is not available, intravenous immune globin given intravenously may be used at a dose of 400 mg/kg.

b. Prophylactic administration of oral acyclovir or valacyclovir beginning 7 days after exposure may also prevent or attenuate varicella disease in healthy children. Prophylactic oral acyclovir or valacyclovir is potentially beneficial for adults, especially those who are immunocompromised or pregnant. Prophylactic dosing of acyclovir is 20 mg/kg per dose, administered 4 times per day with a maximum daily dose of 3,200 mg (e.g., 800 mg PO QID) or valacyclovir 20 mg/kg per dose, administered 3 times per day with a maximum daily dose of 3,000 mg (e.g., 1 gram PO TID). This should be continued for 7 days.

c. Varicella vaccine of susceptible persons administered ideally within 3 days but up to 5 days after exposure (followed by a second dose of vaccine at least 28 days after the first dose in persons 13 years of age or older) may prevent or modify disease.

d. Because vaccine is contraindicated in pregnancy, a pregnant woman with no evidence of immunity (either prior infection or vaccine) with significant varicella exposure is a candidate for acyclovir or valacyclovir prophylactic therapy.

Pre-exposure

a. Varicella vaccine is a live, attenuated viral vaccine that is given subcutaneously as a 2-dose series. For persons 13 years of age or older, the second dose should be given at least 28 days after the first dose. The vaccine should be stored in a frost-free freezer at an average temperature of −15°C (+5°F) or colder.

b. There are two types of varicella vaccines available in the United States: Varivax, which contains only chickenpox virus; and ProQuad, which contains a combination of measles, mumps, rubella, and varicella (chickenpox) vaccines, also called MMRV. ProQuad is only licensed for use in children ages 12 months through 12 years. It can be given to children for their routine 2 doses of chickenpox vaccine at age 12 to 15 months and age 4 to 6 years.

Effectiveness

Effectiveness is 86% against varicella infection and 95% against severe disease after 1 dose, and it is 98% after 2 doses.

Duration of Protection

Appears to be long-lasting after 2 doses (at least 25 years)

Contraindications and Precautions to Varicella Vaccine

Contraindications
1. History of a serious reaction (e.g., anaphylaxis) after a previous dose of varicella vaccine or to a varicella vaccine component
2. Pregnancy currently or in a patient who may become pregnant within 1 month
3. Any malignant condition, including blood dyscrasia, leukemia, lymphoma, or any type of other malignant neoplasm affecting the bone marrow or lymphatic system
4. A patient receiving high-dose systemic immunosuppression therapy (e.g., 2 weeks or more of daily prednisone or equivalent of 20 mg or more [or 2 mg/kg or more for body weight])
5. Family history of congenital or hereditary immunodeficiency in a first-degree relative (e.g., parents, siblings)

when the immunocompetence of the potential vaccine recipient has not been clinically substantiated or verified by a laboratory

6. A child age 1 year or older with CD4⁺ T-lymphocyte percentages less than 15% or a child, adolescent, or adult age 6 years or older with CD4⁺ T-lymphocyte count less than 200 cells per microliter

7. For combination MMRV only (approved only for use in children 1 to 12 years of age), primary or acquired immunodeficiency, including immunosuppression associated with AIDS or other clinical manifestations of HIV infections, cellular immunodeficiency, hypogammaglobulinemia, and dysgammaglobulinemia

8. Use of aspirin or aspirin-containing products to relieve symptoms from chickenpox. The use of aspirin in children with chickenpox has been associated with Reye syndrome, a severe disease that affects the brain and liver and can be fatal. The American Academy of Pediatrics recommends also avoiding treatment with ibuprofen if possible because it has been associated with life-threatening bacterial skin infections. Non-aspirin medications, such as acetaminophen, should be used to relieve fever from chickenpox.

Precautions

1. Recent receipt within the previous 11 months of antibody-containing blood products (specific interval depends on product). People who have received varicella vaccine should not receive blood products for 14 days after vaccination, unless the benefits of the blood product outweigh the need for protection from vaccination.

2. Moderate to severe acute illness with or without fever

Frequently Asked Questions

Can an infant younger than 12 months of age receive the varicella vaccine if they were exposed to the chickenpox or zoster virus?

The minimum age for varicella vaccine is 12 months. Vaccination is *not* recommended for infants younger than 12 months of age, even as post-exposure prophylaxis. A healthy infant should receive no specific treatment or vaccination after exposure to VZV.

Should a dose of varicella vaccine be given to infants younger than 12 months of age if they are traveling internationally?

Varicella vaccine is neither approved nor recommended for children younger than 12 months of age in any situation.

Can the varicella vaccine be used to prevent chickenpox after someone is exposed?

The vaccine has been shown to be effective if given within 3 days of exposure to the varicella virus, and it may be beneficial if given up to 5 days after exposure.

Should a child who had chickenpox prior to their first birthday get the first dose of varicella vaccine at age 1 year?

If the child had confirmed varicella disease or laboratory evidence of prior disease, it is not necessary to vaccinate regardless of age at infection. If there is any question that the illness was actually varicella, the child should be vaccinated.

Is it recommended that children who received one varicella dose 12 years ago at age 1 year be vaccinated with a second dose at this time?
Yes. The current CDC recommendation is for 2 doses of the varicella vaccine regardless of age, for anyone school age and older without evidence of immunity. For everyone whose varicella immunity is based on vaccination, 2 doses of varicella vaccine are recommended.

If a child or adult has not had documented chickenpox but has had shingles, is varicella vaccination still recommended?
No. Shingles is caused by varicella zoster virus, the same virus that causes chickenpox. A history of shingles based on a health care provider diagnosis is evidence of immunity to chickenpox. A person who has had shingles does not need to be vaccinated against varicella.

If a patient has a very mild case of chickenpox (<10 lesions), are they considered immune or should they receive the varicella vaccine?
A case of chickenpox, whether it is mild, moderate, or severe, produces immunity to varicella. A patient with a reliable history of chickenpox does not need to receive the varicella vaccine. However, if there is any doubt about the diagnosis, it is best to vaccinate the patient. There is no harm in vaccinating a patient who may already be immune.

Should an infant receive the varicella vaccine if they are living in a household with a person who is pregnant or someone who is immunocompromised?

Yes. Based on available data, healthy children are unlikely to transmit the vaccine virus, and transmission of vaccine virus to household contacts has rarely been documented. Transmission of the vaccine virus occurs almost exclusively when the vaccinated person develops a rash following vaccination.

What are the recommendations for the use of varicella vaccine in children with HIV or other immunodeficiencies?
The CDC recommends the use of varicella vaccine in children with humoral but not cellular immunodeficiencies. Single antigen varicella vaccine should be considered for HIV-infected children ages 1 to 8 years with $CD4^+$ T-lymphocyte percentages $\geq 15\%$ or for children age 9 years and older with $CD4^+$ T-lymphocyte counts ≥ 200 cells per microliter. Eligible children should receive 2 doses of varicella vaccine with a 3-month interval between doses.

Should health care personnel avoid contact with immunocompromised patients after receiving varicella vaccine?
No. This is not necessary unless the person who was vaccinated develops a rash. If the vaccinated person develops a rash 7 to 21 days following vaccination, they should avoid prolonged close contact with a pregnant or immunosuppressed household contact or patient who is known to be susceptible to varicella, until the rash resolves.

What should be done when hospital employees claim that they have had chickenpox but their varicella antibody titers show no antibodies?

If the health care employee's history of chickenpox cannot be verified, the employee should receive 2 doses of varicella vaccine at least 4 weeks apart.

A health professions student (medical, nursing, dental, physical therapy, etc.) received 2 valid, appropriately spaced, documented doses of varicella vaccine. Subsequently, a titer was drawn for whatever reason, and the titer was negative. Is it recommended to revaccinate this individual with 2 doses of varicella vaccine?
No. Documented receipt of 2 doses of varicella vaccine supersedes the result of subsequent serologic testing. Most commercially available tests for varicella antibody are not sensitive enough to detect vaccine-induced antibody, which is why it is *not* recommended to perform post-vaccination testing.

Is receipt of a single documented dose of zoster vaccine proof of varicella immunity in a health care employee who has no other evidence of immunity?
No. Receipt of zoster vaccine is not proof of prior varicella disease. Per the CDC, acceptable evidence of varicella immunity in health care personnel includes (1) documentation of 2 doses of varicella vaccine given at least 28 days apart, (2) history of varicella or herpes zoster based on physician diagnosis, (3) laboratory evidence of immunity, or (4) laboratory confirmation of disease. If a health care employee has already received a dose of zoster vaccine but has no evidence of immunity to varicella, the zoster dose can be considered the first dose of the 2-dose varicella vaccine series.

How soon after varicella exposure does the varicella vaccine need to be administered if it is used in a post-exposure setting?
Varicella vaccine is effective in preventing chickenpox or reducing the severity of the disease if used within 72 hours (3 days), and possibly up to 5 days, after exposure. Not every exposure to varicella leads to infection, so for future immunity, varicella vaccine should be given, even if more than 5 days have passed since the exposure.

What are the circumstances in which a varicella titer should be obtained after vaccination?
Obtaining post-vaccination serologic testing is *not* recommended in any group, including health care personnel.

Should all pregnant women have serology screening for varicella?
No. Serologic testing for varicella should only be considered for women who do not have evidence of immunity (either a reliable history of chickenpox or documented vaccination). Once a person has been found to be seropositive, it is not necessary to test them again in the future.

What should be done in the situation in which a full-term, healthy, 2-month-old infant was exposed to their mother and another household contact with varicella for the past week?
There is no evidence that healthy full-term infants born to women in whom varicella occurs more than 48 hours after delivery are at increased risk for serious complications from the disease. Varicella zoster immune globulin (VariZIG) can be given up to 10 days after exposure, but it is only recommended

for newborn infants whose mothers have signs and symptoms of varicella around the time of delivery (5 days before to 2 days after), hospitalized premature infants born at 28 or more weeks of gestation whose mothers do not have evidence of immunity to varicella, or hospitalized premature infants born at less than 28 weeks of gestation or who weigh 1,000 grams or less at birth regardless of their mothers' evidence of immunity to varicella. In the above situation, VariZIG would not be recommended. If the infant develops varicella, it would be managed as it would be for any healthy child.

HERPES ZOSTER (SHINGLES)

Did you know that:

- The term *herpes zoster* is derived from the Greek word *herpes*, meaning creeping, and *zoster*, meaning a belt-like binding or girdle that describes a herpes zoster rash encircling the waist.
- Otto von Bismarck ("Iron Chancellor" and architect of the unification of Germany), James H. Doolittle (American aviation pioneer), Golda Meir (fourth prime minister of Israel), Charles Lindbergh ("Lucky Lindy," aviator and explorer), David Letterman (late night TV host), Robin Williams (actor and comedian), Roseann Barr (comedian who described herpes zoster as "worse than labor pains"), and Lin-Manuel Miranda (Broadway writer, producer, and actor) all suffered from severe bouts of herpes zoster (shingles).

Herpes zoster is a neurocutaneous disease caused by the reactivation of the varicella zoster (chickenpox) virus, which has become latent in the dorsal spinal ganglia, and may occur years or decades after primary illness with chickenpox. It is generally associated with normal aging, which is associated with a reduction in cellular immunity, and with anything that causes reduced immunocompetence (e.g., bone marrow and solid organ transplantations, hematologic malignancies, solid tumors, HIV, and immunosuppressive medications). Other risk factors include female gender, White race, trauma, surgery, and persons with early varicella (e.g., varicella in utero or early infancy). Without vaccination, up to one in three persons will develop herpes zoster sometime during their lifetime, with an estimated 1 million cases occurring annually in the United States.

Clinical features include a prodromal illness of headache, photophobia, malaise, fever, and abnormal skin sensation or pain in the affected area. This is followed by the development of the zoster rash that is unilateral involving one to three adjacent dermatomes. Thoracic, cervical, and ophthalmic areas are most commonly involved. The rash initially starts as a painful, erythematous, and maculopapular rash, which then evolves into vesicles over several days before crusting. Full resolution of the rash may take 2 to 4 weeks. Occasionally, the rash does not develop but the patient continues with abnormal skin sensation and pain in the affected area. The pain may be so debilitating that a patient cannot tolerate any touching of the skin, even by the light touch of a tissue.

Complications

a. Postherpetic neuralgia (PHN), the most common complication, develops in 10% to 18% of people, with older age increasing the risk. It ranges from mild to excruciating constant or intermittent pain occurring and persisting after the resolution of the rash. The pain may persist for

weeks, months, or even years, and it may be completely debilitating. Risk factors include age 50 years or older and severe zoster disease. People older than age 80 years are four times more likely to develop neuralgia compared to those younger than age 60 years.
b. Herpes zoster ophthalmicus occurs when herpes zoster presents in the ophthalmic division of the fifth cranial nerve. It occurs in up to 15% of cases and can lead to reduced vision and even blindness. Untreated, 50% to 70% develop acute ocular complications, including acute retinal necrosis. These complications may occur in both immunocompetent and immunocompromised hosts.
c. Secondary infection of the herpes zoster rash, which may lead to permanent scarring or changes in skin pigmentation.
d. Neurologic complications, including encephalitis, ventriculitis, cranial nerve palsies, meningoencephalitis, myelitis, and contralateral ischemic stroke syndrome.
e. Rarely, varicella zoster virus viremia can lead to pneumonia, hepatitis, and disseminated intravascular coagulation.

Transmission

Transmission is person-to-person via direct contact with zoster lesions; however, airborne transmission may occur in certain settings. A person is contagious from the time the rash erupts until the lesions are crusted. Transmission may be decreased by covering the lesions and preventing contact. One cannot develop shingles from contact with a person with shingles. However, if the person never had chickenpox previously, direct contact with a shingles lesion could lead to an initial case of chickenpox (primary varicella zoster infection), and the patient would be susceptible to shingles later in life.

Prevention

a. Herpes zoster vaccine (Shingrix) is an inactivated, subunit, recombinant glycoprotein E adjuvanted vaccine that was licensed in the United States in 2017. It is administered intramuscularly and is routinely recommended for all adults 50 years of age or older **whether or not** they have reported a prior episode of shingles, previously received the live, attenuated varicella vaccine (Zostavax) or the chickenpox vaccine, or had chickenpox in the past. It is given as a 2-dose series with an interval of 2 to 6 months between doses. Shingrix is also recommended for adults 19 years old or older who have weakened immune systems because of disease or therapy. The live, attenuated herpes zoster vaccine (Zostavax) is no longer available in the United States.

Effectiveness

Shingrix provides strong protection against shingles and PHN in all patients 50 years old or older. The efficacy is 96.9% in adults aged 50 to 59 years, 97.4% in adults aged 60 to 69 years, and 91.3% in adults aged 70 years or older. In adults with weakened immune systems, studies show that Shingrix is 68% to 91% effective in preventing shingles, depending on the condition that affects the immune system. The efficacy in the prevention of PHN is high at 91.2% for those older than 50 years of age and 88.8% for those 70 years of age or older.

Duration of Protection

Immunity remains strong for at least 7 years after receiving the 2-dose series. No booster dose of vaccine is recommended at this time.

Contraindications and Precautions to Herpes Zoster Vaccine

Contraindications
1. Severe allergic reaction (e.g., anaphylaxis) after a previous dose or to a vaccine component

Precautions
1. Moderate or severe acute illness with or without fever
2. Experiencing an acute episode of herpes zoster infection. Shingrix is not a treatment for herpes zoster or PHN.

Frequently Asked Questions

Recombinant, adjuvanted zoster vaccine is approved by the FDA for people 50 years of age or older. Does the CDC recommend that health care providers vaccinate people in their 50s?
Yes, the CDC recommends the use of the recombinant, adjuvanted zoster vaccine in people 50 years of age or older to protect against herpes zoster and its complications.

Is there an upper age limit for receipt of the zoster vaccine?
There is no upper age limit for using the recombinant, adjuvanted zoster vaccine. The incidence of herpes zoster increases with increasing age; an estimated 50% of persons living until age 85 years will develop zoster. The CDC recommends the vaccine for everyone aged 50 years or older.

Is it necessary to ask if a person has ever had chickenpox or shingles prior to administering zoster vaccine?

No. All persons aged 50 years or older, whether or not they have a history of chickenpox or shingles, should receive the recombinant, adjuvanted zoster vaccine unless they have a medical contraindication to vaccination. Serologic studies show that almost everyone born in the United States before 1980 has had chickenpox. It is also not recommended or necessary to test for varicella antibody prior to administering the vaccine.

Should a person get the recombinant, adjuvanted zoster vaccine if they already received the live, attenuated zoster vaccine in the past?
Yes, the CDC recommends that all persons 50 years of age or older who had previously received the live, attenuated zoster vaccine in the past receive the recombinant, adjuvanted zoster vaccine. The live, attenuated zoster vaccine was discontinued in the United States in November 2020. It is recommended that one wait at least 8 weeks after the previously received live, attenuated vaccine (if the vaccine was received in another country).

How soon after a case of shingles can a person receive the recombinant, adjuvanted zoster vaccine (Shingrix)?
The general rule for any vaccine is to wait until the patient is over the acute stage of the illness and symptoms have resolved. There is no specific length of time that one needs to wait after having shingles before one can receive the recombinant, adjuvanted zoster vaccine (Shingrix).

What should be done in the situation in which a 60-year-old patient was inadvertently given varicella vaccine instead of zoster vaccine?

If a provider inadvertently administers varicella vaccine to a person for whom zoster vaccine is indicated, the dose should not be considered valid and the patient should be administered a dose of zoster vaccine during the same visit.

If a 65-year-old patient has an underlying condition that requires monthly treatment with intravenous immune globulin (IVIG), can they receive the zoster vaccine?
Yes. The recombinant, adjuvanted herpes zoster vaccine is an inactivated vaccine so there is no concern about interference by circulating antibody in the IVIG with the development of antibodies to this vaccine.

When can a patient who is receiving immunosuppressive chemotherapy receive zoster vaccine?
Adults 19 years old or older who have or will have weakened immune systems because of disease or therapy should receive 2 doses of the recombinant, adjuvanted zoster vaccine (Shingrix). Optimally, they should receive the dose prior to the start of chemotherapy because they will have a better immune response to the vaccine. If needed, people with weakened immune systems can get the second dose 1 or 2 months after the first. If the patient is receiving high-dose steroids, isoantibodies, immune mediators, or immunomodulators, it is recommended to wait 1 month after the therapy is discontinued before administering the recombinant, adjuvanted zoster vaccine so that the person will have a better immune response. If the person is receiving low doses of methotrexate, azathioprine, or 6-mercaptopurine, it is not necessary to wait because these therapies are not considered immunosuppressive.

PNEUMOCOCCAL DISEASE

Did you know that:

- Charles Bronson (actor), James Brown (the "Godfather of Soul"), Leo Tolstoy (author of *War and Peace*), Rene Descartes (French philosopher, mathematician, and scientist), and horror film actor Boris Karloff all died from pneumococcal pneumonia.
- The organism *Streptococcus pneumoniae* was first identified concurrently in 1881 in France by Louis Pasteur and in the United States by George Sternberg.
- Adults 50 years old or older comprise approximately 34% of the population of the United States but account for 92.8% of all the cases of invasive pneumococcal disease.
- In 1911, Sir Almroth Wright, a scientist renowned for his work developing an effective vaccine for typhoid fever, was sent to South Africa to develop and test a pneumococcal vaccine in order to alleviate the burden of epidemic disease in gold miners. Despite vaccinating more than 50,000 miners and claiming his results showed that the vaccine worked, his data did not hold up well to scrutiny. This left him with the unfortunate nickname "Sir Almost Right."

Capsular polysaccharides are an important determinant of pathogenicity and form the basis for classifying pneumococci by serotypes. More than 100 different serotypes have been identified to date.

Since the introduction of routine infant PCV-7 vaccine in 2000 and PCV-13 in 2010, indirect vaccine effects have reduced invasive pneumococcal infections among unvaccinated persons of all ages, including those aged 65 years or older. There were an estimated 17,390 cases and 2,900 deaths occurring among persons of all ages in the United States in 2021; there were 11,887 cases of the invasive pneumococcal disease (IPD) (e.g., pneumonia, bacteremia, meningitis), and 2,349 deaths, with 81% of the deaths occurring in persons older than 50 years of age. Persons 65 years of age or older account for almost 40% of all deaths from IPD.

The conjugate pneumococcal vaccines (PCV7 and PCV13) have had a major impact on the incidence of invasive disease among young children, resulting in a 98% decrease in disease caused by the 13 serotypes in PCV13. This decrease has been offset partially by increases in invasive disease caused by serotypes not included in PCV13. Indirect effects of the conjugate vaccine have reduced invasive pneumococcal infections among unvaccinated persons of all ages. However, pneumococcal pneumonia and IPD remain important causes of illness and death, with an estimated 150,000 hospitalizations annually for pneumococcal pneumonia, more than 1,500 cases of bacteremia with a case fatality rate of 2% to 4% (and up to 60% in the elderly), and 2,000 cases of meningitis with a case fatality rate of 22% in adults and 8% in children. Extended valency pneumococcal conjugate vaccines (PCV15 and PCV20) have been licensed in the United States for use in the adult population (2021) and pediatric population (2022 and 2023).

Transmission

Person to person by respiratory droplet contact. Viral upper respiratory infections, including influenza, can predispose to pneumococcal infection and transmission.

Incubation Period

Varies by type of infection but can be as short as 1 to 3 days. Individuals at increased risk for pneumococcal disease include those with chronic heart disease (especially those with cyanotic heart disease and cardiac failure), chronic lung disease (including asthma, especially if treated with prolonged high-dose oral steroids), diabetes mellitus, cerebrospinal fluid (CSF) leaks, cochlear implant, sickle cell disease and other hemoglobinopathies, chronic or acquired asplenia or splenic dysfunction, HIV infection, diseases associated with treatment with immunosuppressive drugs or radiation therapy (e.g., malignant neoplasms, leukemias, lymphomas, and Hodgkin disease, or solid organ transplantation), congenital immunodeficiency (e.g., B and T lymphocyte deficiency, complement deficiencies [especially C1, C2, C3, and C4 deficiency], phagocyte disorders, alcoholism, chronic liver disease, and cigarette smokers).

Prevention

Pneumococcal vaccine—two types of pneumococcal vaccine available

a. 23-valent polysaccharide vaccine (PPSV23)
b. Pneumococcal protein conjugate vaccines
   i. 15-valent protein conjugate vaccine (PCV15))—each capsular polysaccharide is individually conjugated to a nontoxic variant of diphtheria toxin carrier protein, CRM197.
   ii. 20-valent protein conjugate vaccine (PCV20))—each capsular polysaccharide is individually conjugated to a nontoxic variant of diphtheria toxin carrier protein, CRM197.

PPSV23 contains 23 pneumococcal serotypes that account for 85% to 90% of invasive disease in persons older than 2 years of age. PPSV23 is effective in preventing bacteremia, bacteremic pneumonia, and meningitis, with an efficacy of 56% to 81%. The vaccine does not prevent non-bacteremic pneumonia.

PCV13 contains 13 pneumococcal serotypes that account for 92% of invasive disease in children younger than 5 years of age. PCV13 has been proven effective in preventing bacteremia, pneumonia (with and without bacteremia), meningitis, and otitis media, with an efficacy of 90% to 100% against the various pneumococcal serotypes contained in the vaccine. This was a routinely recommended vaccine of childhood given as a 4-dose series at 2, 4, 6, and 15 to 18 months. Doses routinely may be given up to 5 years of age. Persons between 6 and 18 years of age who are at increased risk for IPD because of functional or anatomic asplenia, sickle cell disease, HIV or other immunocompromising conditions, cochlear implant, or CSF leak were recommended to receive a single dose of PCV13 regardless of whether they had received PPSV23 in the past. Conjugate vaccines such as PCV13 also decrease nasopharyngeal colonization and indirectly reduce the risk of invasive pneumococcal disease in unvaccinated contacts. The expanded valency vaccines PCV15 and PCV 20 have replaced PCV13 in the United States. PCV20 and PCV15 contain 20 and 15 pneumococcal serotypes, respectively, with the additional 7 and 2 serotypes providing coverage for an additional 38.2% and 10.6% of invasive disease, respectively, over PCV13. PCV20 and PCV15 have been proven effective in preventing bacteremia, pneumonia (with and without bacteremia), meningitis, and otitis media, with an efficacy of 90% to 100% against the various pneumococcal serotypes contained in the vaccine. There are currently no studies comparing the efficacy of PCV20 to the PCV15 pneumococcal conjugate vaccine.

Pneumococcal conjugate vaccine is a routinely recommended vaccine of childhood given as a 4-dose series at 2, 4, 6, and 15 to 18 months of age.

PCV15 contains 15 pneumococcal serotypes that include 2 additional serotypes compared to PCV13, which provides a 10.6% increase in coverage of invasive disease caused by these two serotypes in children and a 15% increase in coverage of invasive disease in adults 65 years of age or older.

PCV20 contains 20 pneumococcal serotypes that include 7 additional serotypes compared to PCV13 and 5 additional serotypes compared to PCV15, which provides up to a 40% increase in coverage of disease caused by these additional 5 to 7 serotypes in children and a 27% increase in coverage of invasive disease in adults 65 years of age or older.

The CDC recommends a dose of PCV20 or a dose of PCV15 followed by a dose of PPSV23 in pneumococcal vaccine-naïve persons for

- all adults age 65 years and older; and
- adults age 19 to 64 years with
  - conditions or treatments that affect the immune system (e.g., HIV infection, lymphoma, leukemia, Hodgkin disease, multiple myeloma, generalized malignancy, radiation therapy, and certain long-term corticosteroid use);
  - functional or anatomic asplenia;
  - cochlear implants or CSF leaks;
  - solid organ transplant;
  - congenital or acquired immune deficiencies;
  - diabetes mellitus;
  - chronic heart disease, including congestive heart failure and cardiomyopathies;
  - chronic liver disease;

- chronic lung disease;
- chronic renal disease and renal failure;
- nephrotic syndrome;
- sickle cell disease or other hemoglobinopathies;
- alcoholism; and
- cigarette smoking, including e-cigarettes and vaping.

For adults aged 19 to 64 years:

Persons who are pneumococcal vaccine naïve or whose vaccination history is unknown	Single dose PCV20 OR PCV 15 followed by PPSV23 ≥ 1 year later
Persons who have started their pneumococcal vaccine series with PCV13 but have not received all recommended PPSV23 doses	Single dose PCV20 OR ≥ 1 dose of PPSV23
Persons who have received PPSV23 only	Single dose PCV20 OR Single dose PCV15 If it has been ≥1 year since receiving PPSV23
Persons who are hematopoietic stem cell transplant (HSCT) recipients	Recommended to receive 4 doses of PCV20m starting 3–6 months after HSCT. Administer 3 doses of PCV20, 4 weeks apart. Administer the 4th PCV20 dose ≥6 months after the 3rd dose or ≥ 12 months after HSCT, whichever is later. IF PCV20 not available, give 3 dose PCV15 4 weeks apart, followed by a single dose of PPSV23 ≥ 12 months after HSCT

For adults aged 65 years or older:

Persons who are pneumococcal vaccine naïve or whose vaccination history is unknown	Single dose PCV20 OR PCV 15 followed by PPSV23 ≥ 1 year later
Persons who have started their pneumococcal vaccine series with PCV13 but have not received recommended PPSV23 dose	Single dose PCV20 OR Dose of PPSV23
Persons who have completed their recommended vaccine series with both PCV13 and PPSV23	Shared clinical decision making recommended regarding use of a supplement PCV20 dose

Vaccine Efficacy

PPSV23 in older adults has an efficacy of approximately 75% against invasive pneumococcal disease. PCVs have an efficacy ranging from 75% in adults to 90% in children younger than 5 years of age against invasive pneumococcal disease.

Contraindications and Precautions to Pneumococcal Vaccines

Contraindications
1. For PCV15, PCV20—severe allergic reaction (e.g., anaphylaxis) after a previous dose or to a vaccine component, including to any vaccine containing diphtheria toxoid
2. For PPSV23—severe allergic reaction (e.g., anaphylaxis) after a previous dose or to a vaccine component

Precautions
1. For PCV15, PCV20, and PPSV23—moderate or severe acute illness with or without fever

Frequently Asked Questions

What should be done in the situation in which a 2-month-old was mistakenly given PPSV23 instead of PCV15 or PCV20?
PPSV23 is not effective in infants and children younger than 24 months of age. PPSV23 given at this age should not be considered part of the pneumococcal vaccination series. PCV15 or PCV20 should be administered as soon as possible after the error was discovered.

Which children should receive PPSV23 vaccine (in addition to PCV15 or PCV20)? At what age should they receive PPSV23?
PPSV23 is recommended for children with an immunocompromising condition, functional or anatomic asplenia, and for immunocompetent children with chronic heart disease, chronic lung disease, diabetes mellitus, CSF leaks, or cochlear

implants. One dose of PPSV23 should be administered to children age 2 years or older at least 8 weeks after the child has received the final dose of PCV15 or PCV20. Children with an immunocompromising condition or functional or anatomic asplenia should receive a second dose of PPSV23 5 years after the first PPSV23 dose.

Can PPSV23 be given to a pregnant woman with asthma?
Yes. PPSV23 is recommended in pregnancy if some other risk factor is present (e.g., on the basis of medical, occupational, lifestyle, or other indications). There are no current guidelines for the use of PCV15 or PCV20 in pregnancy.

Given that PPSV23, PCV15, and PCV20 are indicated for smokers aged 19 through 64 years, should adults who use smokeless tobacco products (e.g., chewing tobacco) also be vaccinated?
No. The CDC does not identify people who use smokeless tobacco products or vaping as being at increased risk for pneumococcal disease or as being in a risk group for vaccination.

Is PCV (15, 20) recommended for adults aged 19 through 64 years who smoke?
Yes. PCVs are recommended for adults aged 19 through 64 years who are smokers. Active smoking increases the risk of developing community-acquired pneumonia and invasive pneumococcal disease.

Is obstructive sleep apnea (OSA) a chronic pulmonary disease that would require PPSV23, PCV15, or PCV20 vaccination for adults younger than 65 years of age?

OSA alone is not an indication for vaccination with PPSV23 for persons 2 through 64 years of age. Persons with OSA often have other pulmonary conditions (e.g., chronic obstructive pulmonary disease) that would put them at increased risk for invasive pneumococcal disease, for which they should be vaccinated.

Can PPSV23 and PCV15 be administered at the same office visit?
No. PCV15 and PPSV23 should not be given at the same visit. If PCV15 is indicated, administer it if at least 1 year has passed since the previous dose of PPSV23 or if no doses of PPSV23 have previously been received. Then wait at least 8 weeks for adults with immune compromise and at least 1 year for all other adults to administer PPSV23.

If an adult who is 19 through 64 years of age has already gotten one or more doses of PPSV23, when should they get PCV15 or PCV20, if indicated?
PCV15 or PCV20 should be administered at least 1 year after the previous dose of PPSV23 was administered. For those who require additional doses of PPSV23, the first such dose should be given at least 8 weeks after PCV15 and at least 5 years since the most recent dose of PPSV23.

If a patient has had laboratory-confirmed pneumococcal pneumonia or other invasive pneumococcal disease, do they still need to be vaccinated with PCV15 or PCV20 and/ or PPSV23?
Yes. There are more than 100 known serotypes of pneumococcus. PCV15 contains 15 serotypes, PCV20 contains 20

serotypes, and PPSV23 contains 23 different serotypes. Infection with one serotype does not necessarily produce immunity to other serotypes. Therefore, if a person is a candidate for vaccination, they should receive it even after one or more episodes of invasive pneumococcal disease.

Do patients who were vaccinated with 1 or 2 doses of PPSV23 before age 65 years need an additional dose of PPSV23 or PCV20 at age 65 years or later?
Yes. Patients who received 1 or 2 doses of PPSV23 for any indication at age 64 years or younger should receive an additional dose of PPSV23 or PCV20 vaccine at age 65 years or older if at least 5 years have elapsed since their previous PPSV23 dose.

If an adult aged 65 years or older has already received 1 dose of PCV13 before age 65 years for an appropriate indication, should another dose of PCV (15 or 20) be given at age 65 years?
No. If a dose of PCV13 was already received before age 65 years for an appropriate indication, no additional PCV (15, 20) doses are needed. A dose of PPSV23 should be administered at age 65 years and at least 1 year following the PCV13 dose.

If a patient older than 65 years of age has recently received 1 dose of PPSV23 and is diagnosed with a medical condition that places them at increased risk for pneumococcal disease and its complications, should a second dose of PPSV23 or a dose of PCV20 be given in 5 years because of the underlying medical condition?
No. Individuals who are first vaccinated with PPSV23 at age 65 years or older should receive only 1 dose, regardless of any

underlying medical condition that they may have developed. These individuals should receive a dose of PCV15 or PCV20 at least 1 year after receiving the PPSV23 if they have not received any other PCV dose.

Should the dose of PCV be repeated if given less than 1 year after a dose of PPSV23? If yes, what is the interval between doses?
No, if inadvertently administered sooner than the recommended interval, no repeat dose is recommended. The two vaccines should never be given during the same visit.

If I inadvertently administer PPSV23 less than 8 weeks after PCV13, do I need to repeat the dose of either vaccine?
No. Administration of PPSV23 less than 8 weeks after PCV13 may increase risk for localized reaction at the injection site but remains a valid vaccination and should not be repeated; the PCV13 dose also remains valid and should not be repeated.

How many doses of PPSV23 can an adult get in a lifetime?
Some adults may be recommended to receive up to 3 doses of PPSV23 in a lifetime. Two doses of PPSV23, given 5 years apart, are indicated for adults with functional or anatomic asplenia and immunocompromising conditions before age 65 years. Those adults should then receive a third dose of PPSV23 or a dose of PCV20 at or after age 65 years, as long as it has been at least 5 years since the previous dose.

How many doses of PCVs (15, 20) can an adult get in a lifetime? Who/when?

All adults are recommended to receive 1 dose of PCV15 or PCV20 in a lifetime. If they received a dose of PCV prior to turning age 65 years (due to a medical indication), they are not recommended to receive an additional dose of PCV. The public health benefits of additional PCV doses has not been evaluated.

Can PPSV23 and/or PCV15/PCV20 be administered to patients with multiple sclerosis?
Yes. Multiple sclerosis is not a contraindication to any vaccine, including either of the pneumococcal vaccines.

When should patients (either children or adults) be vaccinated if they are scheduled to have either cochlea implant placement or an elective splenectomy?
It is preferable that the person planning to have the procedure have antibodies to pneumococcus at the time of the surgery. If possible, the appropriate vaccine should be administered prior to the cochlea implant or splenectomy. Infants and children 2 through 71 months of age should continue to receive PCV15 or PCV20 vaccine according to the recommended vaccine schedule.

MENINGOCOCCAL DISEASE

Did you know that:

- The "meningitis belt" refers to a region stretching across sub-Saharan Africa, which has seen recurring epidemics of meningococcal meningitis. An estimated 250,000 people developed meningitis and 25,000 died when the

largest epidemic in recorded history spread through the region in 1996 and 1997. The Meningitis Vaccine Project has provided widespread vaccination with a low-cost conjugate meningococcal type A vaccine, resulting in an 89% decrease in disease and an 83% decrease in deaths from 2009 to 2013.
- In the pre-antibiotic era, the case fatality rate from meningococcal disease was 70% to 85%. Today, despite effective antimicrobial therapy and state-of-the-art intensive care, the overall case fatality rate remains at 10% to 15%.
- Many patients with severe meningococcal sepsis respond poorly to treatment with antimicrobial agents, steroids, or vasopressor agents, and death may occur within hours of onset.
- Patients with meningococcal meningitis who do not develop septic shock are less likely to die; however, they are at risk for developing sensorineural hearing loss, mild to moderate cognitive deficits, or seizure disorders.
- Patients receiving the terminal compliment inhibitors eculizamab or ravulizumab (for treatment of atypical hemolytic uremic syndrome or nocturnal paroxysmal hematuria) have a 1,000-fold to 2,000-fold increased incidence of meningococcal disease.

Meningococcal disease is caused by the organism *Neisseria meningitidis* (encapsulated gram-negative diplococcus), which is strictly a human pathogen. Asymptomatic carriage is common, with 10% of the general population and 25% to 30% of the adolescent/young adult population being carriers. Less than 1% of carriers will become symptomatic with disease. Most common clinical presentations of disease are meningitis, accounting for approximately 50% of the cases with a 3% to 10% fatality rate, and meningococcal sepsis (meningococcemia), accounting for 35% to 40% of cases with up to a 40% fatality rate. Both presentations may be associated with serious permanent sequelae. Fatality rates and rates of serious outcomes are significantly higher in the adolescent and young adult populations compared to the general population (23% vs. 13%). Other clinical presentations that are less common include pneumonia, occult bacteremia, septic arthritis, polyserositis, conjunctivitis, pericarditis, and otitis media.

Onset of disease can be nonspecific but often is abrupt and may progress rapidly over several hours. Patients develop fever; chills; sore throat; nausea and/or vomiting; general aches; diarrhea; headache; malaise; limb pain; abnormal skin color; cold hands and feet; and a rash that initially can be macular, maculopapular, petechial, or purpuric. In fulminant cases, purpura, limb ischemia, coagulopathy, pulmonary edema, shock with poor peripheral perfusion, hypotension, confusion, tachycardia, tachypnea and oliguria, coma, and death may occur in hours despite appropriate therapy. The signs and symptoms of meningitis are indistinguishable from other causes of meningitis.

Complications and Sequelae

a. Meningococcemia: skin scars from necrosis, limb loss from gangrene, renal insufficiency, septic arthritis, pneumonia, epiglottis, pericarditis, death
b. Meningitis: hearing loss, seizures, hemiparesis, spastic quadriplegia, cerebral infarction, cranial nerve palsies, cortical venous thrombophlebitis, cognitive deficits, death

Risk factors for disease include impaired immunity (e.g., terminal complement component deficiency, properdin deficiency, factor

D or factor H deficiencies), functional or anatomic asplenia, nasopharyngeal irritation and disruption of the mucous membranes, and social behaviors that predispose to exposure to secretions. Also at risk are persons traveling to or residing in countries where *N. meningitidis* is endemic; military recruits; persons attending summer camps and colleges who will be living in a dormitory setting; and microbiologists, laboratory personnel, and other health care workers who are routinely exposed to *N. meningitidis*.

Most common serogroups causing disease include A, B, C, Y, X, and W-135. Serogroup distribution varies over time and geographically. The most common serogroups in the United States are B, C, Y, and W135; in Europe, serogroup B; in the African meningitis belt, serogroups A and X; in Saudi Arabia, serogroup W-135; and in New Zealand, serogroup B.

Transmission

Person to person through contact with droplets from the respiratory tract. Transmission requires close contact. Close contact is defined as follows:

a. Household contact, especially children younger than 2 years of age
b. Child care or preschool contact at any time during 7 days before onset of illness
c. Direct exposure to index patient's secretions through kissing or through sharing toothbrushes or eating utensils, markers of close social contact, at any time during 7 days before onset of illness
d. Mouth-to-mouth resuscitation, unprotected contact during endotracheal intubation at any time 7 days before onset of illness

e. Frequently sleeping in same dwelling as index patient during 7 days before onset of illness
f. Passengers seated directly next to the index case during airline flights lasting more than 8 hours

Incubation Period

Incubation period is 1 to 10 days but usually less than 4 days.

Prevention

Post-exposure

a. Antibiotic chemoprophylaxis—**regardless of immunization status**, close contacts of all persons with invasive meningococcal disease are at high risk and should receive post-exposure chemoprophylaxis (Table 12). Chemoprophylaxis ideally should be initiated within 24 hours after the index patient is diagnosed; prophylaxis given more than 2 weeks after exposure has little value.
b. Quadrivalent meningococcal conjugate vaccine (MenACWY) should be given **in addition** to antibiotic chemoprophylaxis to those persons who have not previously been immunized. Vaccine is given intramuscularly.

Pre-exposure

a. Quadrivalent meningococcal conjugate vaccine (MenACWY)—routinely recommended vaccination for all adolescents 11 to 18 years of age, persons with HIV, and persons 2 to 54 years of age with persistent complement component deficiency or functional or anatomic asplenia (Table 13). Vaccine should also be given to other persons

Table 12 MENINGOCOCCAL CHEMOPROPHYLAXIS

Antibiotic	Dose	Duration	Cautions
Rifampin	10 mg/kg PO q 12 hours (max 600 mg)	2 days	Can interfere with efficacy of oral contraceptives and some seizure and anticoagulant medications. Not recommended to be used in pregnant women.
Ceftriaxone			
<15 years of age	125 mg IM	Single dose	
≥15 years of age	250 mg IM	Single dose	
Ciprofloxacin	20 mg/kg PO (max 500 mg)	Single dose	Not recommended to be used in pregnant women.
Azithromycin	10 mg/kg PO (max 500 mg)	Single dose	Not routinely recommended.

Table 13 SCHEDULE FOR ROUTINE DOSING OF ADOLESCENTS WITH MENINGOCOCCAL VACCINE

Initial (Primary) Dose	Booster Dose
11–12 years (preferred timing)	16 years
13–15 years	16–18 years
≥16 years	No booster needed

at increased risk for meningococcal disease (see above risk factors for disease).

Routine 2-dose primary series administered 2 months apart for persons 2 to 54 years of age with persistent complement component deficiency, functional or anatomic asplenia, and adolescents and adults with HIV infection. A booster dose should be given every 5 years.

A dose should be given to persons traveling to or residing in countries where *N. meningitidis* is endemic; military recruits; persons attending summer camps and colleges who will be living in a dormitory setting; and microbiologists, laboratory personnel, and other health care workers who are routinely exposed to *N. meningitidis*. A booster dose may be given every 5 years if the person continues to be in situations of increased risk.

Vaccination with a meningococcal conjugate vaccine is recommended for infants aged 2 through 23 months at increased risk for meningococcal disease. Infants at increased risk for meningococcal disease are

- those with persistent complement component deficiencies (C3, C5–C9, properdin, factor D, and factor H);
- those with functional or anatomic asplenia (including sickle cell disease);
- healthy infants in communities with a meningococcal disease outbreak for which vaccination is recommended; and
- those traveling to or residing in areas where meningococcal disease is hyperendemic or epidemic.

Table 14 shows the available meningococcal conjugate vaccines.

Table 14 CURRENTLY AVAILABLE MENINGOCOCCAL CONJUGATE VACCINES

Vaccine	Trade Name	Type of Vaccine	Meningococcal Serogroups Covered
MPSV4	Menomune	Polysaccharide	A, C, W, Y
MenACWY	Menactra	Conjugate	A, C, W, Y
MenACWY-CRM	Menveo	Conjugate	A, C, W, Y
Hib-MenCY-TT	MenHibrix	Conjugate	C, Y (and *Haemophilus influenzae* type b [Hib])
Men ABCWY	Penbraya	Conjugate and recombinant protein	A, B, C, W, Y

b. Meningococcal serogroup B vaccine (MenB)—currently has a category B recommendation, which means that the MenB vaccine series may be administered to adolescents and young adults aged 16 to 23 years to provide short-term protection against most strains of serogroup B meningococcal disease based on the clinical judgment of the health care provider for the individual patient (weighing the risks and benefits) and shared clinical decision-making between the health care provider and the patient. The preferred age for MenB vaccination is 16 to 18 years.

Two MenB vaccines are licensed in the United States. MenB vaccine should be administered as either a 2- or 3-dose series of MenB-FHbp (Trumenba) or a 2-dose series of MenB-4C (Bexsero). The two MenB vaccines are not interchangeable; the same vaccine product must be used for all doses. Both vaccines may be administered concomitantly with other vaccines indicated for this age group.

MenB-FHbp (Trumenba)—the 2-dose series is recommended for healthy adolescents and adults given at 1 and 6 months; the 3-dose series is recommended for persons at increased risk for meningococcal disease and is given at 0, 2, and 6 months.

MenB-4C (Bexsero)—2-dose series given at least 1 month apart.

    a. Pentavalent meningococcal conjugate vaccine (MenABCWY)—active immunization of individuals 10 through 25 years of age against invasive meningococcal diseases caused by *N. meningitidis* serogroups A, B, C, W, and Y. Administer 2 doses at least 6 months apart for prevention of meningococcal disease caused by serogroups A, B, C, W, and Y. Administer 1 dose for prevention of meningococcal disease caused by serogroups A, C, W, and Y. A booster dose may be administered to individuals who have previously completed a primary series with MenABCWY or MenB-FHbp vaccine or who have previously received MenACWY conjugated vaccines.

Efficacy

MenACWY—80% to 100% for the serotypes contained in the vaccine

MenB—50% to 80%

MenABCWY—80% to 98% for the serotypes contained in the vaccine

Duration of Immunity

For MCV4 vaccines, duration of immunity is thought to be 3 years. Duration of immunity for MenB vaccines is thought to be 1 or 2 years. For MCV5, duration of immunity is unknown at this time but is thought to be similar to MCV4 for ACWY components and similar to MenB vaccine for the B component.

Contraindications and Precautions to Meningococcal Vaccines

Contraindications
1. Severe allergic reaction (e.g., anaphylaxis) after a previous dose or to a vaccine component

Precautions
2. Moderate or severe acute illness with or without fever

Frequently Asked Questions

Who is recommended to be vaccinated against meningococcal disease?
MCV4 is recommended for

- all children and teens, aged 11 through 18 years of age;
- people younger than 22 years of age if they are or will be a first-year college student living in a residential hall;
- people aged 2 months or older with functional or anatomic asplenia (MenHibrix may be used for children aged 6 weeks through 18 months in this group—vaccine only contains meningococcal serogroups C and Y);

- people aged 2 months or older who reside in or travel to certain countries in sub-Saharan Africa as well as to other countries for which meningococcal vaccine is recommended (e.g., travel to Mecca, Saudi Arabia, for the annual Hajj); and
- microbiologists who work with meningococcus bacteria in the laboratory.

MenB is recommended for

- people 10 years of age or older who have functional or anatomic asplenia;
- people 10 years of age or older who have persistent complement component deficiency or are at risk during an outbreak caused by a vaccine serogroup; and
- microbiologists who work with meningococcus bacteria in the laboratory.

MenABCWY is recommended for

- individuals 10 through 25 years of age.

Can adolescents receive quadrivalent meningococcal vaccine and serogroup B meningococcal vaccine at the same time?
Yes. Meningococcal and other vaccines may be administered during the same visit but at a different anatomic site if feasible.

Is meningococcal vaccination recommended for adolescents during outbreaks?
Yes. If a meningococcal disease outbreak is serogroup A, C, W, or Y, vaccination with quadrivalent meningococcal vaccine is

recommended for adolescents identified as being at increased risk. If the meningococcal disease outbreak is serogroup B, adolescents identified as being at increased risk because of the outbreak should be vaccinated with serogroup B meningococcal vaccine.

Why isn't it recommended to administer the serogroup B meningococcal vaccine to all adolescents?

Administration of the serogroup B meningococcal vaccine to patients 16 through 23 years of age is left to the discretion of the clinician and shared decision-making with the patient. Detailed efficacy and safety data for making policy recommendations are not yet available because these vaccines were licensed for use in the United States under an accelerated approval process. And the current burden of disease with this serotype is low. In the setting of an outbreak of serogroup B disease, vaccination would be appropriate.

How many doses of serogroup B meningococcal vaccine are necessary?

Both serogroup B meningococcal vaccines require more than 1 dose for maximum protection: 2 doses of MenB-4C (Bexsero) (0, ≥1 month after first dose) and 2 doses of MenB-FHbp (Trumenba) for healthy adolescents and young adults (0 and 6 months) or 3 doses of Trumenba (0, 2 months after first dose, 6 months after first dose) for adolescents and young adults with underlying conditions that place them at risk for meningococcal disease. The same vaccine product must be used for all doses.

Are there any groups for whom a booster dose of MenB vaccine is recommended after completion of the primary series?

Yes. A booster dose of MenB vaccine is recommended for persons with functional or anatomic asplenia, with the first booster dose given 1 year after completion of primary series and then every 2 or 3 years thereafter.

Should persons with continued high risk of meningococcal disease receive additional doses of meningococcal vaccine beyond the 3- or 5-year booster?
Yes. People should receive additional booster doses (every 5 years) if they continue to be at highest risk for meningococcal infection.

HUMAN PAPILLOMAVIRUS

Did you know that:

- Infection with human papillomavirus (HPV) is universal among humans (both females and males).
- The vast majority of U.S. teenagers are not aware that a single sexual contact with an infected partner with or without a visible lesion can spread HPV.
- Every 20 minutes in the United States, a person acquires an infection with HPV.
- In the United States, among girls 14 to 19 years old, HPV incidence has dropped by 88% since the introduction of HPV vaccines in 2006. For women 20 to 24 years old, the rate is down by 81%.

In the United States, HPV will infect 80% of sexually active males and females in their lifetime. According to the CDC, there are approximately 13 million new genital HPV infections in the

United States each year, 75% of which occur in people aged 15 to 25 years. For most people, HPV clears spontaneously, but for those who do not clear the virus, infection can lead to significant cancers and other diseases in men and women. There is no way to predict who in the population will clear the virus, although the oncogenic types are more likely to persist and lead to the development of malignancy than the benign types.

HPV causes a range of disease manifestations, including cutaneous nongenital warts of the skin (e.g., common skin warts, plantar warts, flat warts, and filiform warts), mucous membranes (e.g., anogenital, oral, nasal, and conjunctival areas), and the respiratory tract (e.g., respiratory papillomatosis). It also is associated with cervical, anogenital, and oropharyngeal dysplasias (precancers) and cancers. More than 100 different serotypes of HPV have been identified. These serotypes are subdivided into high-risk, oncogenic serotypes and low-risk, non-oncogenic serotypes. The most common high-risk serotypes include types 16, 18, 31, 33, 35, 39, 45, 51, 52, 56, 58, 59, 68, 69, 73, and 82, which account for 98% of all cervical cancers. Serotypes 16 and 18 account for 70% of all cervical cancers and the vast majority of other anogenital cancers. The most common low-risk serotypes include types 6, 11, 40, 42, 43, 44, and 54, with serotypes 6 and 11 accounting for 90% of all external anogenital warts.

Transmission

Transmission takes place person-to-person by close contact. Nongenital warts are acquired through contact with HPV and minor trauma to the skin. Anogenital HPV infection is the most common sexually transmitted infection in the United States. Most infections are subclinical and resolve spontaneously within 2 years. Persistent infection with high-risk serotypes is associated with development of cervical, vulvar, vaginal, penile, anal, and oropharyngeal cancers. In the case of respiratory papillomatosis, infection is transmitted to an infant through the birth canal during delivery by aspiration of infectious secretions. The finding of genital warts or laryngeal lesions in young children should raise the suspicion of child abuse.

Incubation Period

Incubation period is unknown but is estimated to range from 3 months to 10 years.

Prevention

Condoms, both male and female, provide some protection, but because the male condom only covers the shaft of the penis, there is still the potential for contact and spread from the anogenital area. Female condoms that cover much of the anogenital area and the entire vagina should provide more protection; however, the usage of female condoms is not widespread.

The best protection is provided by HPV vaccines.

Post-exposure
　a. HPV vaccine—there is only one HPV vaccine currently available in the United States:
　　i. HPV9 (contains 9 serotypes—6, 11, 16, 18, 31, 33, 45, 52, and 58. It is licensed for use in *both* females and males aged 9 to 45 years. It is recommended as a 2-dose series 6-12 months apart in persons ages 9-14 years and a 3-dose series given over 6 months in persons 15-26 years old.
　　ii. HPV vaccine is still recommended to be given after onset of sexual activity and even if known to be

HPV-positive because subsequent infection with other serotypes is possible.
   iii. The vaccine is *not* a therapeutic vaccine and is not useful in treating any specific HPV-related conditions.

Pre-exposure
  a. HPV vaccine—the best time to administer is prior to the onset of sexual activity. It is not prudent to give the vaccine based on perceived risk because it is not possible to predict onset of sexual activity in any patient. In multiple studies in New Zealand, Australia, and the United States, there was no increased sexual activity related to immunizing adolescents with HPV vaccine.
     i. HPV9 (contains 9 serotypes—6, 11, 16, 18, 31, 33, 45, 52, and 58. Licensed for use in both females and males aged 9 to 45 years. It is given as a 2- or 3-dose intramuscular series at 0, 1 or 2, and 6 months.
     ii. Vaccines are *not* recommended to be used as therapeutic vaccines.

Immunogenicity

  a. HPV9 vaccine is 98% to 100% effective for the prevention of cervical precancers due to vaccine serotypes and prevention of vulval intraepithelial neoplasia and vaginal intraepithelial neoplasia.
  b. HPV9 vaccine is 90% effective for the prevention of genital warts and anal cancers.

The vaccination rate in females and males 13 to 17 years of age in the United States overall is 62.6% when receiving all 3 doses. Young patients are strongly encouraged to be vaccinated, and parents should be strongly encouraged to have their children vaccinated. The emphasis must be "this is a cancer vaccine" not a "sexual activity" vaccine. The recommendation of the health care provider is the most important factor in a patient's or parent's acceptance of the vaccination.

Duration of Immunity

Duration is at least 12 years.

Contraindications and Precautions to HPV Vaccine

Contraindications
1. Severe allergic reaction (e.g., anaphylaxis) after a previous dose or to a vaccine component
2. Severe allergic reaction (e.g., anaphylaxis) to yeast

Precautions
1. Moderate or severe acute illness with or without fever
2. Pregnancy

Frequently Asked Questions

If a person was vaccinated at age 11 years and completed the 3-dose series, and is now aged 20 years and sexually active, should she receive a booster dose of vaccine?
No. Long-term studies have shown no loss of efficacy at least 13 years after the first series of vaccinations.

Should individuals who have completed a 3-dose series of HPV2 or HPV4 receive a booster dose or be revaccinated with a 3-dose series of HPV9?

At this time, there are no recommendations for a booster dose of vaccine or revaccination with HPV9. There are data that indicate revaccination with HPV9 after a series of HPV4 is safe. Clinicians should decide if the benefit of immunity against five additional oncogenic strains of HPV is justified for their patients.

If a patient received 1 or 2 doses and has not completed the 3-dose series, should the series be restarted?
No. Even if a long period of time has passed since the last vaccine dose, the series should not be restarted but, rather, should be resumed where it was left off and can be completed at any time. However, if multiple doses are needed, the timing between doses cannot be shortened.

Will giving HPV vaccination encourage sexual activity in my teenage child?
No. Multiple studies have shown no difference in the initiation of sexual activity in adolescents who have or have not received the HPV vaccine. These studies used sexually transmitted disease incidence, use of contraception, pregnancy, and abortion rates in determining the lack of differences in the two groups.

If a woman becomes pregnant and has received only 1 or 2 doses of HPV vaccine, can she complete the series during the pregnancy?
No. Even though HPV vaccine poses no risk to the fetus, the doses should be delayed until after the pregnancy. She may receive the vaccine even if she is breastfeeding.

If a patient has received 1 or 2 doses of HPV2 or HPV4 vaccine, can the patient complete the series with HPV9?

Yes. Any available HPV vaccine may be used to continue to complete the series for females. HPV4 or HPV9 can be used to continue or complete the series for males. However, receiving fewer than 3 doses of HPV4 or HPV9 may provide less protection against genital warts caused by HPV types 6 and 11 than the usual 3-dose series. There are no data on the efficacy of the five additional HPV types included in HPV9 if the person receives fewer than 3 doses.

Can the HPV vaccine damage a woman's ovaries?
No. The CDC and FDA have found no evidence that HPV vaccine is associated with premature ovarian failure. There has also been no evidence of amenorrhea or irregular menses in women who have received the vaccine.

Why is HPV vaccine recommended if Pap tests can detect cervical cancer?
Pap tests are effective screening tests and can detect precancerous changes before progression to cancer. But the vaccine actually prevents cancer in the first place, and Pap tests are not perfect (overall 50% sensitivity), and not all women get tested as often as recommended.

Should women still have Pap tests done after receiving HPV vaccine?
Yes. Although the HPV9 vaccine protects against more than 90% of the cancer-producing HPV viruses, many women have received either the HPV2 or HPV4 vaccines, which protect against approximately 70% of oncogenic virus types. Pap screening recommendations may well change as a higher percentage of women are vaccinated.

Do women and men whose sexual orientation is same sex need HPV vaccine?
Yes. HPV vaccine is recommended for females and males regardless of their sexual orientation.

Is there an accelerated vaccination schedule to complete the HPV vaccine series?
No. There is no accelerated schedule for completing the HPV vaccine series. The recommended schedule of 0, 1 or 2, and 6 months should be followed.

If HPV vaccine is inadvertently given subcutaneously instead of intramuscularly, does the dose need to be repeated?
Yes. No data exist on the efficacy or safety of HPV vaccine given by the subcutaneous route; therefore, the CDC and the manufacturers recommend that a dose of HPV vaccine given by any route other than intramuscular should be repeated. There is no minimum interval between the invalid subcutaneous dose and the repeat dose.

HEMOPHILUS INFLUENZAE TYPE B DISEASE

Did you know that:

- Before the availability of *Hemophilus influenzae* type b (Hib) conjugate vaccine, each year in the United States approximately 20,000 children younger than 5 years of age got Hib disease, and 3% to 6% died from their disease.
- The bacterium was first isolated by Richard Pfeiffer from the sputum of patients in 1892 during an outbreak of

influenza, and it was proposed that there was a causal association between the bacteria and the clinical syndrome of influenza.

Hemophilus influenzae type b (Hib) is a pleomorphic gram-negative coccobacillus. It may cause a variety of different infections, including pneumonia, bacteremia, meningitis, epiglottis, septic arthritis, osteomyelitis, cellulitis, otitis media, purulent pericarditis, endocarditis, endophthalmitis, peritonitis, and gangrene. Before the introduction of effective Hib conjugate vaccines (before 1990), Hib was the most common cause of bacterial meningitis in children in the United States. There were 20,000 cases a year of invasive disease, with the peak age of infections occurring in infants between 6 and 18 months of age. Non-type b encapsulated strains cause disease similar to type b infections. Non-typeable strains commonly cause infections of the respiratory tract (e.g., otitis media, sinusitis, pneumonia, and conjunctivitis). Less commonly, these strains may cause bacteremia, meningitis, chorioamnionitis, and neonatal sepsis.

Unimmunized children 4 years of age or younger are at increased risk of invasive Hib disease. Other risk factors that predispose to invasive disease in all ages include sickle cell disease, asplenia, HIV infection, certain immunodeficiency syndromes, and malignant neoplasms. Historically, invasive Hib disease was more common in boys; Black, Alaskan Native, Apache, and Navajo children; day care attendees; children living in crowded conditions; and children who were not breastfed. Since the introduction of Hib conjugate vaccines in the United States, the incidence of invasive Hib disease has decreased by 99%. Currently, invasive disease occurs primarily in unimmunized or underimmunized children and among infants too young to have completed the primary immunization series. Hib remains a major pathogen in many resource-limited countries where Hib vaccine is not routinely available. In the United States, non-typeable and non-type b *H. influenzae* now causes the majority of invasive disease in all age groups.

Transmission

The major reservoir of Hib is young infants and toddlers who carry the organism in the upper respiratory tract, which is the natural habitat of *H. influenzae* in humans. Transmission is person-to-person by inhalation of respiratory tract droplets or by direct contact with infected respiratory tract secretions. In neonates, infection is acquired intrapartum by aspiration of amniotic fluid or by contact with genital tract secretions containing the organism. Pharyngeal colonization by *H. influenzae* is common, especially with non-typeable and non-type b capsular types.

Incubation Period

Unknown

Prevention Is Available Only for *Hemophilus influenzae* Type b

Post-exposure
Careful observation of exposed, unimmunized, or incompletely immunized children who are household, child care, or nursery school contacts of patients with invasive Hib disease is essential.

Chemoprophylaxis—the risk of invasive Hib disease is increased among unimmunized or incompletely immunized household contacts younger than 4 years of age. Rifampin (20 mg/

kg, max dose 600 mg—given once a day for 4 days) eradicates Hib from the pharynx in approximately 95% of carriers and decreases the risk of secondary invasive infection in exposed household contacts. Nursery and child care center contacts younger than 4 years of age may also be at increased risk of secondary disease. The following are indications for rifampin chemoprophylaxis for contacts of index cases of invasive Hib disease:

- For all household contacts (defined as people living with the index patient or nonresidents who spend 4 or more hours with the index patient for at least 5 of the 7 days preceding the day of hospital admission) in the following circumstances:
  - Household with at least one contact younger than 4 years of age who is unimmunized or incompletely immunized
  - Household with a child younger than 12 months of age who has not completed the primary Hib series
  - Household with a contact who is an immunocompromised child, regardless of that child's Hib immunization status
- For preschool and child care contacts when two or more cases of Hib invasive disease have occurred within 60 days.
- For index patient, if younger than 2 years of age or member of household with a susceptible contact and **treated with a regimen other than ceftriaxone or cefotaxime**, chemoprophylaxis is provided just before hospital discharge.

Hib vaccine—in addition to chemoprophylaxis, unimmunized or incompletely immunized children should receive a dose of Hib vaccine and should be scheduled for completion of the recommended age-specific immunization schedule.

Pre-exposure
Hib vaccine—vaccine is given intramuscularly.

  i. Primary series—depending on the vaccine used, the recommended primary series consists of 3 doses given at 2, 4, and 6 months of age (DTaP-IPV/PRP-T) or 2 doses given at 2 and 4 months of age (PRP-OMP, PRP-OMP-HepB). If PRP-OMP vaccine is **not administered** as both doses in the primary series, a third **dose of Hib conjugate vaccine is needed** to complete the primary series.
  ii. Booster dose—recommended to be given at 12 through 15 months of age.

Contraindications and Precautions to Hib Vaccine

Contraindications
1. Severe allergic reaction (e.g., anaphylaxis) after a previous dose or to a vaccine component
2. Age younger than 6 weeks

Precautions
1. Moderate or severe acute illness with or without fever

Efficacy

Efficacy is 98% to 100% against Hib.

Frequently Asked Questions

Can all the licensed Hib-containing vaccines be used interchangeably?

Yes, but there is one exception. The GSK monovalent product (Hiberix) is only licensed for the booster dose of vaccine.

If Hiberix is inadvertently given as some or all of the doses of the primary Hib vaccine series, do the doses need to be repeated?
No, the administered doses count and *do not* need to be readministered with another Hib vaccine.

If an infant received 1 dose of Hib at 4 months of age, and another at 16 months of age, do they need any additional doses of Hib vaccine?
No. If an infant receives a dose of Hib vaccine at 15 months of age or older, they do not need any further Hib vaccine doses regardless of the number of doses received before 15 months of age.

If a 4-year-old patient received dose number 3 of Hib vaccine at 6 months of age, does the child need a fourth dose of Hib?
Yes. All children younger than 5 years of age need at least 1 dose of Hib vaccine on or after the first birthday. The last dose should be separated from the previous dose by at least 2 months.

The booster dose of Hib vaccine is recommended to be given at 12 to 15 months of age. Is it necessary to administer the booster dose 2 months later, if a patient received their first dose of Hib vaccine at 12 months of age?
If the child received a primary series (2 or 3 doses) of Hib vaccine in the first year of life, then the final (booster) dose of the series may be given as early as 12 months, provided at least 2 months have passed since the last dose. An

unvaccinated 12- to 14-month-old child should receive 1 dose of Hib vaccine as the primary series and a booster dose 2 months later. Unvaccinated children 15 to 59 months of age need only a single dose of any licensed conjugate Hib vaccine.

Does an 8-year-old who does not have a record of ever receiving Hib vaccine need a dose?
The CDC does not recommend routine Hib vaccination of healthy children aged 59 months or older, even if they have no prior history of receiving Hib vaccination.

Which adults should receive a dose of Hib vaccine?
Hib vaccine is recommended for adults with sickle cell disease, leukemia, HIV infection, and persons with functional or anatomic asplenia if they have not previously received Hib vaccine. A standard pediatric dose of any Hib vaccine may be used. Hib vaccine is not routinely recommended for healthy adults 19 years of age or older.

When should Hib vaccine be administered to a person having a splenectomy?
When elective splenectomy is planned, vaccination with pneumococcal, meningococcal, and Hib vaccines should be administered at least 2 weeks prior to the surgery, if possible. If the vaccines are not administered before surgery, they should be administered as soon as the person's condition stabilizes postoperatively.

POLIOVIRUS INFECTIONS

Did you know that:

- None of the three strains of wild poliovirus can survive outside the human body for very long and will die out if the virus cannot find an unvaccinated person to infect.
- Franklin Delano Roosevelt, the 32nd president of the United States, contracted paralytic polio at the age of 39 years, resulting in partial paralysis of his legs and the inability to walk without the aid of crutches or leg braces.
- In addition to Franklin D. Roosevelt, a well-known polio survivor, others include science fiction writer Arthur C. Clarke, artist Frida Kahlo, golfer Jack Nicklaus, swimmer (and actor) Johnny Weissmuller, actors Mia Farrow and Alan Alda, and singer/songwriters Neil Young and Joni Mitchell.
- Poliomyelitis has affected humankind since ancient times. An Egyptian monument from the 18th dynasty (1403–1365 BC) depicts a crippled young man with a withered and shortened right leg, with his foot held in a typical equinus position characteristic of flaccid paralysis.
- In the pre-vaccine era, poliomyelitis was the leading cause of permanent disability. It was a feared disease because it could strike anyone, and no means existed to protect oneself or one's children.
- Epidemic poliomyelitis in the early 20th century was associated with a high case fatality rate of 27.1%.
- The first iron lung was constructed in 1928, and its widespread use in the 1930s and 1940s rapidly decreased the case-fatality ratio of bulbar forms of poliomyelitis.

- The game Candy Land was invented in 1948 by a patient trying to cheer up kids in a polio ward.
- Polio can be completely eradicated with the use of vaccine.

Polioviruses are group C RNA enteroviruses that include serotypes 1, 2, and 3. Poliovirus infections occur only in humans. Approximately 72% of poliovirus infections in susceptible children are asymptomatic. A nonspecific febrile illness with low-grade fever and sore throat occurs in 24% of people who become infected. Aseptic meningitis (pleocytosis with a lymphocytic predominance), sometimes with paresthesias, occurs in 1% to 5% of patients a few days after the minor illness has resolved. Paralytic polio occurs in less than 1% of infected persons. This presents as the rapid onset of asymmetric acute flaccid paralysis with areflexia of the involved limb and residual paralytic disease which occurs in approximately two-thirds of people with acute motor neuron disease. Cranial nerve involvement and paralysis of respiratory tract muscles can occur.

Adults who contracted paralytic poliomyelitis during childhood may develop the non-infectious post-polio syndrome 15 to 40 years later. Post-polio syndrome is characterized by slow and irreversible exacerbation of weakness occurring in the muscle groups involved during the original infection. It is thought to be due to physiologic attrition of motor units already less innervated as a result of the earlier acute infection. Muscle and joint pain is common. Studies estimate the risk of post-polio syndrome in poliomyelitis survivors to be 25% to 40%.

No cases of polio have originated in the United States since 1979; the last case of wild-type polio in a U.S. resident traveling abroad occurred in 1986, and the last imported case of polio in the United States occurred in 2023. Globally, polio cases have decreased by more than 99% since 1988 due to a concerted global effort to eradicate the disease. In 1994. the World Health Organization (WHO) Region of the Americas was certified polio-free, followed by the WHO Western Pacific Region in 2000, the WHO European Region in June 2002, and the WHO South East Asian Region in 2014. Of the three types of wild poliovirus, type 2 wild poliovirus transmission has been successfully eradicated since 1999. In 2023, only 2 countries continued to have endemic circulating wild-type poliovirus—Afghanistan and Pakistan—down from 125 countries in 1988. However, as long as wild-type poliovirus continues to circulate, children in all countries are at risk of contracting polio.

Transmission

Spread is by the fecal, oral, and respiratory routes. Infection is more common in infants and young children and occurs at an earlier age among children living in poor hygienic conditions. Communicability of poliovirus is greatest shortly before and after the onset of clinical disease, when the virus is present in the throat and is excreted in high concentration in the feces. Virus persists in the throat for approximately 2 weeks after onset of illness and is excreted in the feces for 3 to 6 weeks. Patients are potentially contagious as long as fecal excretion persists.

Incubation Period

For nonparalytic polio, the incubation period is 3 to 6 days. For the onset of paralysis in paralytic poliomyelitis, the incubation period is usually 7 to 21 days.

Prevention

Pre-exposure Prophylaxis

a. Inactivated polio vaccine (IPV)—4 doses of IPV vaccine are recommended for routine immunization of all infants and children.

　i. The first 2 doses of the 4-dose vaccine series should be given at 2-month intervals beginning at 2 months of age (2 and 4 months). The third dose is recommended to be given at 6 through 18 months of age. A fourth and final dose in the series should be administered at 4 years of age or older, regardless of the number of previous doses and at a minimum interval of 6 months from the third dose. If a child misses an IPV dose at 4 through 6 years of age, the child should receive a booster dose as soon as feasible.

　ii. Most adults living in the United States are presumed to be immune as a result of previous immunization. However, immunization is recommended for certain adults who are a greater risk of exposure to wild-type polioviruses than the general population, including the following:

- Travelers to areas or countries where poliomyelitis is or may be epidemic or endemic
- Laboratory workers handling specimens that may contain wild-type polioviruses
- Health care personnel in close contact with patients who may be excreting wild-type polioviruses

For unimmunized or incompletely immunized adults, primary immunization with IPV vaccine is recommended as a series of 3 doses. Two doses of IPV vaccine should be given at intervals of 1 or 2 months (4 to 8 weeks); a third dose is given 6 to 12 months after the second dose. If 3 doses of IPV cannot be administered within the recommended intervals before protection is needed, the following alternatives are recommended:

- If >8 weeks are available before protection is needed, 3 doses of IPV should be administered ≥4 weeks apart.
- If <8 weeks but >4 weeks are available before protection is needed, 2 doses of IPV should be administered ≥4 weeks apart.
- If <4 weeks are available before protection is needed, a single dose of IPV is recommended.

Vaccine Efficacy

Both IPV and oral live, attenuated polio vaccine (OPV) are highly immunogenic and effective in preventing poliomyelitis. IPV is the only polio vaccine available in the United States. After 2 doses of IPV, greater than 95% of recipients seroconvert to the 3 polio serotypes contained in the vaccine. After 3 doses, seroconversion is seen in 99% to 100% of vaccine recipients.

Duration of Immunity

At least 18 years after a 3-dose series of vaccine

Contraindications and Precautions to Polio Vaccine

Contraindications
Vaccine is contraindicated for people who have experienced an anaphylactic reaction after a previous dose of IPV vaccine or to streptomycin, neomycin, or polymyxin B.

Precautions
1. Moderate or severe acute illness with or without fever
2. Pregnancy, although there is no evidence that IPV vaccine causes harm to pregnant individuals or their fetuses

Frequently Asked Questions

If there is no longer any polio in the Western Hemisphere, why do we still recommend universal polio vaccination?
If polio vaccination were discontinued in the United States, there would be millions of susceptible children within a year. Because wild polio infection still occurs in the world, the virus could be imported and an epidemic could result.

After what age is routine polio vaccine no longer recommended?
Routine polio vaccination is not recommended for persons 18 years of age or older who reside in the United States. Exceptions include adults at risk for exposure to poliovirus: traveling in polio-endemic areas of the world (currently Afghanistan or Pakistan), working in a laboratory and handling specimens that might contain polioviruses, and those who may have close contact with someone who could be infected with poliovirus.

Is vaccine-derived poliovirus a risk in the United States?
Vaccine-derived poliovirus (VDPV) is a strain of poliovirus that was initially contained in OPV and that has mutated over time and behaves more like the wild-type virus. These strains may be transmitted to unvaccinated persons and cause illness, including paralytic poliomyelitis—indistinguishable from the illness caused by wild-type poliovirus. VDPV can cause

outbreaks in countries where vaccine coverage with OPV is low. Because OPV has not been used in the United States since 2000 and vaccine coverage with IPV is high, the risk of VDPV in the United States is very low. It would be possible for an unvaccinated person to acquire VDPV from someone who recently received live oral vaccine in another country.

How long is OPV virus shed in the stool after the dose?
OPV may be shed in the stool for up to 6 weeks, but it can be longer in immunosuppressed individuals. Viral shedding in the stool is generally longest following the first dose and is generally shorter with each subsequent dose.

A 4-year-old entering pre-kindergarten has a vaccination record that shows that they received 4 doses of IPV given at 2 months, 4 months, 6 months, and 2 years of age. Does this child need a booster dose of vaccine?
Yes. The current recommendations are that a child receive 4 doses of IPV vaccine, with the last dose being given on or after the fourth birthday.

If a 10-year-old child adopted from another country received 3 doses of OPV before their first birthday, should they receive an additional dose of IPV?
Yes. The patient should receive a dose of IPV now. The final dose of the polio vaccine series should be received on or after the fourth birthday, regardless of the number of doses received prior to the fourth birthday.

What polio vaccination schedule should be used for older children who have not completed their IPV series?

The schedule for polio vaccination for unvaccinated or undervaccinated older children through age 17 years is a total of 3 doses of IPV: 2 doses of IPV separated by 4 to 8 weeks, and a third dose 6 to 12 months after the second dose. Polio vaccine is not routinely administered to persons 18 years of age or older.

Should adults get vaccinated against polio if they are traveling to a high-risk area where polio still occurs?
If an adult at increased risk previously received only 1 or 2 doses of polio vaccine (either OPV or IPV), they should receive the remaining dose(s) of IPV regardless of the interval since the last polio vaccine dose. If the at-risk adult previously completed a primary course of polio vaccine (3 of more doses of OPV or IPV), they may be given another dose of IPV to ensure protection. Only "one" 1 booster dose of polio vaccine in a person's lifetime is recommended. It is not necessary to administer a booster dose each time a person travels to an area where polio may be occurring.

Should an adult who was diagnosed with polio as a child and has some residual effects and who will be traveling to a high-risk area where polio still occurs be vaccinated with polio vaccine even though they had polio in the past?
Immunity to one of the serotypes of polio does not produce significant immunity to the other serotypes. A history of having recovered from polio disease should not be considered evidence of immunity to polio. In this situation, it is appropriate to vaccinate this person with a dose of IPV if they are traveling to a high-risk area.

A 22-year-old patient has been accepted to a medical school that requires polio vaccine for all the students. The patient had 2 documented doses of OPV vaccine as a child and then received a dose of IPV upon college entry at age 18 years. How many additional doses of IPV should this patient receive to complete the series and on what schedule?

Persons who receive a mixed series of OPV and IPV should receive a total of 4 doses of vaccine. The dose of IPV can be counted as the third dose in the primary series. The minimum interval between the third and last doses in the polio vaccination series is 6 months; therefore, the final dose in the series should be administered 6 months or longer after the last IPV dose.

ROTAVIRUS INFECTIONS

Did you know that:

- Worldwide, rotavirus is estimated to cause 450,000 to 600,000 deaths in children each year, which is approximately 20% to 25% of the estimated 1.9 million annual deaths from diarrhea.
- Rotavirus diarrheal illness causes 1,200 to 1,600 deaths per day in developing countries.
- Fluid loss from severe rotavirus diarrhea in an infant can be as much as 20 mL/kg per hour.

Rotaviruses are segmented, double-stranded RNA viruses with at least seven distinct antigenic groups (A through G). Group A viruses are the major causes of rotavirus diarrhea worldwide. Serotyping is based on the two surface proteins, VP7 glycoprotein

(G) and VP4 protease-cleaved hemagglutinin (P). Prior to introduction of the rotavirus vaccine, G types 1 through 4 and 9 and P types 1A and 1B were the most common in the United States. Rotavirus infection is the leading cause of severe acute diarrhea among young children worldwide. In the United States, prior to the introduction of rotavirus vaccine in 2006, rotavirus caused an estimated 20 to 60 deaths, 55,000 to 70,000 hospitalizations, 205,000 to 272,000 emergency department visits, and 410,000 outpatient visits annually. Nearly every child in the United States was infected with rotavirus by 5 years of age, and most developed gastroenteritis. Rotavirus was responsible for 5% to 10% of all gastroenteritis episodes among children younger than 5 years of age in the United States.

Infection begins with the acute onset of fever and vomiting, followed 24 to 48 hours later by watery diarrhea. Symptoms generally persists for 3 to 8 days. In moderate to severe cases, dehydration, electrolyte abnormalities, and acidosis may occur. The epidemiology of rotavirus disease in the United States has changed dramatically since rotavirus vaccines became available in 2006. The overall burden of rotavirus disease has significantly declined. In the first 2 years after the RV5 vaccine became available, emergency room visits and hospitalizations for rotavirus decreased by 85% (estimated 40,000 to 60,000 fewer gastroenteritis hospitalizations among children younger than 5 years of age). There were also substantial reductions in office visits for gastroenteritis during this time.

Transmission

Fecal–oral route. Rotavirus is present in high titers in the stool of infected persons several days before and may continue up to 10 days after onset of clinical disease. Only a small inoculum

(100 colony-forming units/gram) is needed for transmission. It can remain viable for weeks to months on contaminated environmental surfaces (e.g., toys and hard surfaces in child care centers), indicating that fomites may also serve as a mechanism of transmission. Respiratory transmission may play a minor role in disease transmission.

Incubation Period

Usually less than 48 hours

Prevention

Pre-exposure
- a. Rotavirus vaccine—there are two rotavirus vaccines licensed for use among infants in the United States (Table 15). In February 2006, a live, oral human–bovine reassortant pentavalent rotavirus vaccine (RV5) was licensed as a 3-dose series for use among infants in the United States. In April 2008, a live, oral human attenuated monovalent rotavirus vaccine (RV1) was licensed as a 2-dose series for infants in the United States. Vaccine is administered orally.
    - i. Rotavirus vaccine can be administered concurrently with other childhood vaccines.
    - ii Preterm infants may be immunized if they are at least 6 weeks of postnatal age and are clinically stable. They should be immunized on the same schedule and with the same precautions recommended for full-term infants. The first dose of the vaccine should be given at the time of discharge or after the infant has been discharged from the nursery.

Table 15 ROTAVIRUS VACCINES

Recommendation for Use	RV5 (RotaTeq—Merck)	RV1 (Rotarix—GSK)
Number of doses in the series	3	2
Recommended ages for doses	2, 4, and 6 months of age	2 and 4 months of age
Minimum age for first dose	6 weeks of age	6 weeks of age
Maximum age for first dose	14 weeks, 6 days of age	14 weeks, 6 days of age
Minimum interval between doses	4 weeks	4 weeks
Maximum age for last dose	8 months, 0 days of age	8 months, 0 days of age

iii. Breastfeeding infants should be immunized according to the same schedule as non-breastfed infants.

iv. Infants who have had rotavirus gastroenteritis before receiving the full series of rotavirus immunization should begin or complete the schedule following the standard age and interval recommendations.

Vaccine Contraindications

1. Rotavirus vaccine should *not* be given to infants who have a history of a severe allergic reaction (e.g., anaphylaxis) after a previous dose of rotavirus vaccine or to a vaccine component. Latex rubber is contained in the RV1 vaccine oral applicator, so infants with a severe allergy to latex (e.g., anaphylaxis) should not receive RV1.

2. Severe combined immunodeficiency and a history of intussusception are contraindications for use of both RV1 and RV5 rotavirus vaccines.

Vaccine Efficacy

RV5—effectiveness after 3-dose series ranges from 96% to 100% against severe rotavirus disease, from 78% to 100% against disease requiring hospitalization, and it is 96% in preventing disease requiring an outpatient visit.

RV1—effectiveness after 2-dose series ranges from 76% to 89% against rotavirus disease requiring hospitalization, and it is 50% in preventing disease requiring an outpatient visit.

Frequently Asked Questions

How long is a person with rotavirus diarrhea contagious?
Infected persons shed large quantities of virus in their stool beginning 2 days before the onset of diarrhea and for up to 10 days after onset of symptoms. Rotavirus may be detected in the stool of persons with immune deficiency for more than 30 days after infection.

Can a person get rotavirus disease more than once?
Yes. A person may develop rotavirus disease more than once because there are many different rotavirus types, but second infections tend to be less severe than the first infections. After a single natural infection, 40% of children are protected against a subsequent rotavirus illness. Persons of all ages can get repeated rotavirus infections, but symptoms may be mild or not occur at all in repeat infections.

Can adults be infected with rotavirus?
Yes. Rotavirus infection of adults is usually asymptomatic but may cause diarrheal illness. Outbreaks of diarrheal illness caused by rotavirus have been reported, especially among elderly persons living in retirement communities and nursing homes.

Should an infant who has already been infected with rotavirus still be vaccinated?
Yes. Infants who have recovered from a rotavirus infection may not be immune to all of the virus types present in the vaccine. So infants who have previously had rotavirus disease should still complete the vaccine series if they can do so by age 8 months.

If it is unknown which rotavirus vaccine an infant previously received, how should the vaccine schedule be completed?
If the product used for a previous dose is unknown, and the infant is at an age when the vaccine can still be administered, a total of 3 doses of rotavirus vaccine should be given. All doses of vaccine should be administered by age 8 months and 0 days. Series may be completed with the vaccine that is available.

If the first dose of rotavirus vaccine is inadvertently given to an infant aged 15 weeks or older, should the vaccine series be continued?
Infants for whom the first dose of rotavirus vaccine was inadvertently administered at age 15 weeks or older should receive the remaining doses of the series at the routinely recommended intervals. The timing of the first dose should not affect the safety and efficacy of the remaining doses. Rotavirus

vaccine should not be given after 8 months, 0 days, even if the series is incomplete.

In the situation in which an infant received the first dose of rotavirus vaccine but got laboratory-confirmed rotavirus disease prior to the second vaccine dose, should the infant complete the vaccine series?
The CDC recommends that infants who have had rotavirus gastroenteritis before receiving the full series of rotavirus vaccination should still start or complete the schedule according to the age and interval recommendations because the initial rotavirus infection might provide only partial protection against subsequent rotavirus disease.

If an infant regurgitates or vomits during or after rotavirus vaccine administration, should the dose be repeated?
No. If an infant spits, regurgitates, or vomits during or after rotavirus vaccine has been administered, the dose should not be repeated. The next dose of vaccine should be administered at the appropriate interval.

Can an infant receive rotavirus vaccine if there are pregnant or immunocompromised individuals who live in the same household?
Infants living in households with pregnant women or immunocompromised people *can* be immunized with rotavirus vaccine. Transmission of vaccine virus strains from vaccines to unimmunized contacts is uncommon.

CONTRAINDICATIONS AND PRECAUTIONS TO COMMONLY USED VACCINES

Table 16 lists the contraindications and precautions to commonly used vaccines.

Table 16 CONTRADICTIONS AND PRECAUTIONS TO COMMONLY USED VACCINES

Vaccine	Contraindications	Precautions
For **all** the vaccines	Severe allergic reaction (e.g., anaphylaxis) after a previous dose or to a vaccine component	Moderate or severe acute illness with or without fever

In addition to the above, additional contraindications and precautions for specific vaccines

Vaccine	Contraindications	Precautions
Diphtheria, tetanus, pertussis (DTaP, DTP) Tetanus, diphtheria, pertussis (Tdap) Tetanus, diphtheria (DT, Td)	For pertussis-containing vaccines: encephalopathy (e.g., coma, decreased level of consciousness, prolonged seizures) not attributable to another identifiable cause within 7 days of administration of a previous dose of DTP, DTaP, or Tdap	GBS within 6 weeks after a previous dose of tetanus toxoid-containing vaccine

History of Arthus-type hypersensitivity reactions after a previous dose of tetanus or diphtheria toxoid-containing vaccine; defer vaccination until at least 10 years have elapsed since the last tetanus toxoid-containing vaccine |

(continued)

Table 16 CONTINUED

Vaccine	Contraindications	Precautions
		For pertussis-containing vaccines: progressive or unstable neurologic disorder (including infantile spasms for DTaP), uncontrolled seizures, or progressive encephalopathy until a treatment regimen has been established and the condition has stabilized
		For DTaP/DTP only
		Temperature of 105°F or higher (40.5°C or higher) within 48 hours after vaccination with a previous dose of DTP/DTaP
		Collapse or shocklike state (i.e., hypotonic hyporesponsive episode) within 48 hours after receiving a previous dose of DTP/DTaP
		Seizure within 3 days after receiving a previous dose of DTP/DTaP
		Persistent, inconsolable crying lasting 3 or more hours within 48 hours after receiving a previous dose of DTP/DTaP
Haemophilus influenzae type b (Hib)	Age younger than 6 weeks	—

Table 16 CONTINUED

Vaccine	Contraindications	Precautions
Hepatitis B	—	Infants weighing less than 2,000 grams (4 lbs, 6.4 oz.)
Human papillomavirus (HPV)	Severe allergic reaction (e.g., anaphylaxis) to yeast—HPV4, HPV9 Severe allergic reaction (e.g., anaphylaxis) to latex—HPV2	Pregnancy
Inactivated poliovirus vaccine (IPV)	—	Pregnancy
Influenza, inactivated injectable (IIV)	Severe allergic reaction (e.g., anaphylaxis) to prior dose of vaccine or to vaccine component	History of GBS within 6 weeks of previous influenza vaccination Persons who experience only hives with exposure to eggs may receive recombinant influenza vaccine (RIV) or, with additional safety precautions, IIV.
Influenza, recombinant (RIV)—Flublok	Severe allergic reaction (e.g., anaphylaxis) after a previous dose or to a vaccine component; RIV does not contain any egg protein, thimerosal, antibiotics, latex, gelatin, or formaldehyde	History of GBS within 6 weeks of previous influenza vaccination

(continued)

Table 16 CONTINUED

Vaccine	Contraindications	Precautions
Influenza, live, attenuated (LAIV)	People younger than age 2 years or older than age 49 years Concomitant use of aspirin or aspirin-containing medication in children or adolescents through age 17 years Specific populations: pregnant women; immunosuppressed people; children aged 2 through 4 years who have asthma or had wheezing within the past 12 months; people who have taken influenza antiviral medications (amantadine, rimantadine, zanamivir, or oseltamivir) within the previous 48 hours: Avoid using these antiviral agents for 14 days after vaccination	History of GBS within 6 weeks of previous influenza vaccination Asthma in persons aged 5 years or older Other chronic medical conditions (other chronic lung diseases; chronic cardiovascular diseases excluding isolated hypertension; diabetes; chronic renal or hepatitis disease; hematologic disease; neurologic disease; and metabolic disorders)

ROUTINE VACCINES FOR VACCINE-PREVENTABLE DISEASES

Table 16 CONTINUED

Vaccine	Contraindications	Precautions
Measles, mumps, rubella (MMR)—live	Known severe immunodeficiency (e.g., from hematologic and solid tumors, receipt of chemotherapy, congenital immunodeficiency, or long-term immunosuppressive therapy, or patients with HIV infection who are severely immunocompromised) Pregnancy	Recent (within 11 months) receipt of antibody-containing blood product (specific interval depends on product) History of thrombocytopenia or thrombocytopenia purpura Need for tuberculin skin testing (Measles vaccine may suppress tuberculin reactivity temporarily. MMR may be administered on the same day as tuberculin skin testing; however, if testing cannot be performed at the same time, the test should be postponed for at least 4 weeks after MMR vaccination.)
Pneumococcal conjugate (PCV)	Severe allergic reaction (e.g., anaphylaxis) to any vaccine containing diphtheria toxoid	—
Rotavirus—live, attenuated oral RV5—RotaTeq RV1—Rotarix	SCID History of intussusception	Immunodeficiency other than SCID Chronic gastrointestinal disease Spina bifida or bladder exstrophy

(continued)

Table 16 CONTINUED

Vaccine	Contraindications	Precautions
Varicella (Var)—live	Known severe immunodeficiency (e.g., from hematologic and solid tumors, receipt of chemotherapy, congenital immunodeficiency, or long-term immunosuppressive therapy, or patients with HIV infection who are severely immunocompromised)	Recent (within 11 months) receipt of antibody-containing blood product (specific interval depends on product) Receipt of specific antivirals (e.g., acyclovir, famiciclovir, or valacyclovir) 24 hours before vaccination; avoid use of these antiviral drugs for 14 days after vaccination
	Pregnancy	

GBS, Guillain-Barré syndrome; SCID, severe combined immunodeficiency.

COVID-19

Did you know that:

- The COVID-19 pandemic has caused more than 700 million cases and 7 million deaths, ranking it as the fifth deadliest pandemic in history.
- Infectivity can begin 4 or 5 days before the onset of symptoms and continue for up to 10 days after the onset of symptoms.
- Up to 40% of infected individuals do not experience symptoms; nevertheless, they can transmit infection and have

viral loads that are equivalent to those of individuals who are symptomatic.
- The virus can live up to 24 hours on cardboard and 2 or 3 days on plastic and stainless steel. Nevertheless, transmission via fomites has not been a significant driver of disease spread.

COVID-19 is caused by SARS-CoV-2 (severe acute respiratory syndrome coronavirus 2), a novel coronavirus first discovered in Wuhan, China, in December 2019. Many early cases were linked to persons who had visited the Huanan Seafood Wholesale Market there, but it is possible that human-to-human transmission started earlier. COVID-19 symptoms range from asymptomatic to fever, sore throat, cough, and fatigue. Loss of taste and smell may occur. Complications include pneumonia, acute respiratory distress syndrome, respiratory failure, septic shock, and death. Cardiovascular complications can include heart failure, myocardial infarction, arrhythmias, venous thromboembolism, and stroke. Disease in children may be complicated by multisystem inflammatory syndrome.

Transmission

SARS-CoV-2 is believed to have originated from bats or a closely related mammal. Virus particles are spread via droplets or aerosols from the respiratory tract of persons with active infection. Despite evidence of survival of virus on surfaces, fomites do not appear to be an important mode of transmission.

Incubation Period

2 to 14 days; typically, 4 to 6 days

Prevention

An array of first-generation SARS-CoV-2 vaccines have helped bring the COVID-19 pandemic under control. In the United States, COVID-19 vaccination is recommended for all persons 6 months of age or older. Globally, more than 50 vaccine candidates have been approved. Some of the more notable COVID-19 vaccines include the following:

mRNA vaccines
　Spikevax (Moderna), Comirnaty (Pfizer–BioNTech)
Recombinant spike protein nanoparticle
　Covovax, Nuvaxovid (Novavax)
Non-replicating viral vector vaccines
　Jcovden (Johnson & Johnson [J&J]/Janssen); Vaxzevria, Covishield (AstraZeneca); Convidecia; Sputnik V
Inactivated virus vaccines
　CoronaVac, Covaxin

Almost all COVID-19 vaccines demonstrated significant protection against the original strain and subsequent variants of concern and were well tolerated. Comirnaty (Pfizer–BioNTech), Spikevax (Moderna), and Sputnik V after 2 doses had the highest efficacy (>90%) in preventing symptomatic cases in clinical trials. As the SARS-CoV-2 pandemic has evolved, COVID vaccines have been less effective in preventing infection with newer viral strains/variants, but they have continued to demonstrate significant ongoing protection against severe disease, hospitalization, and death. Vaccination has also demonstrated benefit in reducing the risk of multisystem inflammatory syndrome in children and post-COVID-19 syndrome or "long COVID." As of 2023, 70% of the world population had received at least 1 dose of a COVID-19 vaccine.

Adverse Events

Swelling, redness, and pain at the injection site are common. Side effects such as fever, chills, tiredness, and headache are common within 7 days of getting vaccinated but are typically mild. These symptoms are more common after the second dose of a Pfizer–BioNTech, Moderna, or Novavax COVID-19 vaccine.

Anaphylaxis is rare (<1 in 100,000 doses), and all patients with anaphylaxis after the first dose of a COVID vaccine who were given a second dose received it without fatality.

There is a rare risk of myocarditis and pericarditis associated with mRNA COVID-19 vaccination, especially among young males. It has most commonly occurred 2 or 3 days after a second dose of mRNA vaccination. Cases of myocarditis and pericarditis have also been reported in people who received Novavax COVID-19 vaccine. In one study, among 18- to 29-year-olds in the United States, myocarditis was reported in an estimated 22 excess cases per 1 million vaccine recipients after the second dose of the Pfizer–BioNTech vaccine and 31 cases per 1 million after the second dose of the Moderna vaccine. Patients with myocarditis typically presented with chest pain, elevated cardiac troponin levels, ST elevations on electrocardiogram, and cardiac magnetic resonance imaging suggestive of myocarditis. Almost all patients recovered with or without treatment. The risk of myocarditis may be further reduced with a longer interval between the first and second dose in the primary series. Of note, the risk of myocarditis after COVID-19 illness (146 per 100,000) is significantly higher than the risk after vaccination. When myocarditis cases after the first and second dose are added together, the risk of it occurring is still almost six times lower than the risk of myocarditis after COVID-19 infection.

Thrombosis with thrombocytopenia syndrome (blood clots with low platelets) was reported following vaccination with the J&J/Janssen COVID-19 vaccine, especially in women younger than 50 years of age (7 per 1 million vaccinated women aged 18 to 49 years). The J&J/Janssen COVID-19 vaccine is no longer available in the United States. An 11- to 21-fold increased risk of Guillain–Barré syndrome was reported after J&J/Janssen COVID vaccination, but no increased risk has been reported following vaccination with Pfizer–BioNTech or Moderna COVID vaccines.

Vaccine Inequity

Vaccine inequity became especially apparent during the COVID-19 pandemic and vaccine rollout. Through 2023, more than 70% of the world population has received at least 1 dose of a COVID-19 vaccine, but only 33% of people in low-income countries have received at least 1 dose. An estimated 50% of COVID-related deaths worldwide could have been averted in lower middle- and low-income countries if those countries had the same access to COVID-19 vaccines as high-income countries. In the United States, Black and Hispanic persons were less likely than Whites to have received a COVID-19 vaccine over the course of the vaccination rollout—a contributing factor to disparities in health outcomes. These disparities have narrowed over time and reversed for Hispanic persons.

Contraindications and Precautions to COVID-19 Vaccines

Contraindications
1. History of a severe allergic reaction (e.g., anaphylaxis) after a previous dose or to a component of the COVID-19

vaccine. (Do not vaccinate with the same COVID-19 vaccine type. May administer the alternate COVID-19 vaccine type.)

Precautions

1. History of a non-severe, immediate (onset less than 4 hours) allergic reaction after administration of a previous dose of one COVID-19 vaccine type (may administer alternate COVID-19 vaccine type)
2. History of a diagnosed non-severe allergy to a component of the COVID-19 vaccine (may administer alternate COVID-19 vaccine type)
3. Moderate or severe acute illness, with or without fever (Defer vaccination until the illness has improved.)W
4. History of multisystem inflammatory syndrome in children (MIS-C) or multisystem inflammatory syndrome in adults (MIS-A) (Delay COVID-19 vaccination—at a minimum—until clinical recovery has been achieved, including return to baseline cardiac function, and it has been at least 90 days after the diagnosis of MIS-C or MIS-A.)
5. History of myocarditis or pericarditis within 3 weeks after a dose of any COVID-19 vaccine (A subsequent dose of any COVID-19 vaccine should be avoided.)

Frequently Asked Questions

Does COVID-19 vaccination cause viral mutation?
COVID-19 vaccines do not cause new variants. New variants of the COVID-19 virus happen because the virus that causes COVID-19 constantly changes through a natural ongoing process of mutation.

Is post-exposure vaccination for COVID-19 effective?
COVID-19 vaccines are not recommended for post-exposure prophylaxis, but individuals with a known or potential SARS-CoV-2 exposure may receive vaccine if they do not have symptoms consistent with COVID-19.

Are COVID-19 vaccines safe in pregnancy?
Maternal vaccination during pregnancy has been shown to be safe and effective, and it protects infants younger than age 6 months from severe COVID-19 and hospitalization. Maternal vaccination is strongly recommended by the CDC and ACOG.

Does COVID vaccination cause infertility?
COVID-19 vaccines will not affect fertility.

Can mRNA COVID vaccines alter one's DNA?
COVID-19 vaccines do not alter DNA. The vaccine mRNA never comes into contact with a person's DNA, which is located in the nucleus of a cell.

Are there potentially harmful ingredients in COVID-19 vaccines?
None of the COVID-19 vaccines contain ingredients such as preservatives, tissues (e.g., aborted fetal cells), antibiotics, food proteins, medicines, latex, or metals.

How do you explain the high rate of adverse events following COVID-19 vaccination reported to the Vaccine Adverse Event Reporting System (VAERS)?
Not all events reported to VAERS are caused by vaccination. Reports of adverse events to VAERS following vaccination,

including deaths, do not necessarily mean that a vaccine caused a health problem.

RESPIRATORY SYNCYTIAL VIRUS

Did you know that:

- Respiratory syncytial virus (RSV) was discovered in 1956. It was isolated from chimpanzees that were suffering with symptoms of a respiratory illness and was originally named chimpanzee coryza agent (CCA). In 1957, this virus was identified in children who also were suffering with respiratory illnesses that were indistinguishable from CCA, and the virus was renamed RSV.
- Humans are the only known reservoir for RSV.
- RSV gets its name from the formation of large cells known as syncytia when infected cells fuse.

RSV is also known as human respiratory syncytial virus or human orthopneumovirus. It causes acute respiratory tract infections in people of all ages and is one of the most common diseases of early childhood. RSV is an enveloped, nonsegmented, negative, single-stranded RNA virus. Almost everyone will be exposed to the virus by age 2 years, with persons of all ages being at risk for repeated infections throughout the lifespan. Reinfection in people older than age 60 years results in up to 10,000 deaths per year in the United States. Severe RSV lower respiratory tract infection resulting in hospitalization most commonly occurs in infants younger than 6 months of age, in premature infants, and in persons 60 years of age and older. Infections in infants and older adults with other medical conditions are at the highest risk for severe disease. The highest risk patients are premature infants; people of all ages with compromised immune systems; young children with congenital heart disease, chronic lung disease, and neuromuscular disorders; and adults aged 60 years or older, particularly those with heart or lung disease. It occurs in annual epidemics generally beginning in the fall and continuing through early spring in temperate climates.

RSV is often divided into two antigenic subtypes (A and B) based on two surface proteins. These subtypes tend to co-circulate at the same time during RSV season. The RSV envelope contains three surface glycoproteins: glycoprotein G, fusion protein F, and a small hydrophobic protein SH. Antibodies directed against F and G are protective and are neutralizing antibodies. The fusion protein F is conserved, making it a perfect target for vaccine and monoclonal antibody development.

There are other viruses found to infect animals that show similarities to RSV. Bovine RSV, found in cows, shares 80% of the genome with human RSV. Bovine RSV also shows a greater risk for causing severe disease in young cattle.

Transmission

Humans are the only source of RSV infection. RSV is transmitted by direct or close contact with contaminated secretions, which may occur when an infected host coughs or sneezes. Viral droplets are transmitted from a cough or sneeze when the droplets land in a person's eyes, mouth, or nose. Transmission can also occur from touching an object with the active virus. RSV can survive for several hours on hard inanimate surfaces and for 30 minutes or more on hands.

Incubation Period

The incubation period for RSV ranges from 2 to 8 days, with 4 to 6 days being the most common time.

Clinical Course

Most often, RSV will result in a mild, upper respiratory viral illness, but in more severe cases, it can cause bronchiolitis and pneumonia. In infants younger than age 6 months, common symptoms include irritability, decreased activity and appetite, mild cough, and apneic episodes of more than 10 seconds. Fever may or may not be present. Almost 2% of children younger than age 6 months with RSV infection may need to be hospitalized. When hospitalized, they often require supplemental oxygen, intravenous fluids, and occasionally mechanical ventilation.

When adults get an RSV infection, symptoms are usually similar to those for other viral upper respiratory infections, with rhinorrhea, anorexia, malaise, and cough. RSV can exacerbate congestive heart failure, asthma, or chronic obstructive pulmonary disease. Older adults are hospitalized with RSV at a rate of approximately 160,000 per year in the United States, with up to 10,000 fatalities annually.

Treatment

There are no specific available treatments that shorten the course of RSV infection or hasten the resolution of symptoms. Management of hospitalized persons with severe RSV is supportive and may include oxygen supplementation, intravenous fluids, careful assessment of respiratory status, and mucus suctioning.

Prevention

Passive Immunization

Nirsevimab (Beyfortus) is a long-acting human recombinant monoclonal antibody that is an RSV F protein-directed fusion inhibitor designed to bind to the fusion protein on the surface of the RSV virus to prevent severe RSV in infants. It is indicated for all infants younger than 8 months of age prior to or during their first RSV season. It is given as a single intramuscular injection (50 mg for infants ≤5 kg; 100 mg for infants >5 kg) and is recommended to be given after birth prior to hospital discharge or during the first week of life, if possible. Duration of protection after the single dose is at least 5 months. A second dose (200 mg administered as two 100-mg injections given at the same time at different injection sites) may be given to infants and children aged 8 to 19 months who are at increased risk of severe RSV disease and entering their second RSV season. This includes children with chronic lung disease of prematurity who required medical support any time during the 6-month period before the start of the second RSV season, children who are severely immunocompromised, children with cystic fibrosis who have manifestations of severe lung disease or weight-for-length less than the 10th percentile, and American Indian or Alaska Native children.

Palivizumab (Synagis) is a humanized monoclonal immunoglobulin G1K antibody directed against a conserved epitope of an antigenic site of the fusion protein F approved to prevent severe RSV in infants and children at high risk for complications. Palivizumab is indicated for children born at less than 32 weeks of gestation who are less than 6 months of age at the onset of the RSV season, children 2 years of age or younger requiring treatment for bronchopulmonary dysplasia within the past 6 months, and children 2 years of age or younger with hemodynamically significant congenital heart disease. It is administered as a monthly intramuscular injection during RSV season.

Active Vaccination

Two vaccines are available to prevent RSV infections. Both are administered as a single dose preferably prior to the start of RSV season, but they may be administered during RSV season.

1. RSVPreF3 (GlaxoSmithKline)—adjuvanted (ASO1E) recombinant prefusion F protein (preF) vaccine. Recommended only for all adults aged 75 years or older and adults aged 60-74 years at increased risk of severe RSV disease.
   Vaccine efficacy against RSV-associated lower respiratory tract disease:
   - 82.6% for season 1
   - 56.1% for season 2
   - Combined season 1 and 2 efficacy: 74.5%
2. RSVpreF (Pfizer)—recombinant preF vaccine. Recommended for use in both older adults aged 60 years or older and pregnant women (administered between 32 and 36 weeks of gestation).
   Vaccine efficacy against RSV-associated lower respiratory tract disease in older adults:
   - 88.9% for season 1
   - 78.6% for season 2
   - Combined season 1 and 2 efficacy: 84.4%
   Vaccine efficacy against RSV-associated lower respiratory tract disease in pregnant women and their infants:
   - 81.8% against severe medically attended lower respiratory tract illness due to RSV in infants from birth through the first 90 days of life

- 69.4% vaccine efficacy through the first 6 months of life in infants
- 57.1% against severe medically attended lower respiratory tract illness due to RSV in mothers from birth through the first 90 days of life
- 51.3% vaccine efficacy through the first 6 months of life in mothers

Contraindications and Precautions

Contraindications
1. Vaccine is contraindicated for people who have experienced an anaphylactic reaction after a previous dose of RSV vaccine or to vaccine component.

Precautions
1. Moderate or severe acute illness with or without fever

Frequently Asked Questions:

How do people get infected with RSV?
RSV is a very common virus that spreads easily between people. It is usually spread via airborne drops from coughing or sneezing. It can survive on hard surfaces for many hours. There is a higher chance of exposure to this virus if one is in an area that has a high density of people.

How can I protect my newborn baby from infection?
Pregnant women should get vaccinated with RSV vaccine between 32 and 36 weeks of gestation. If the baby is born within 2 weeks of the mother receiving the vaccine, the mother's vaccine status is unknown, or the mother did not receive

RSV vaccine, then all infants younger than 8 months of age can receive a dose of nirsevimab (extended-duration monoclonal antibody). The recommended time to administer this dose is after birth prior to hospital discharge or during the first week of life during RSV season; otherwise, all infants younger than 8 months of age can receive a dose at the start and during their first RSV season. Other commonsense measures include keeping the newborn baby away from anyone with a cough or other cold-like symptoms, making sure that everyone who touches the newborn washes their hands first, and limiting the time that infants spend at child care centers. Be mindful that babies also get infected when older siblings carry the virus home. Wash your baby's clothes, toys, and bedding frequently. Clean and disinfect potentially contaminated surfaces regularly, and keep your baby away from crowds and young children.

Can RSV infect a person more than once?
People frequently experience multiple RSV infections during their life. People usually produce antibodies against RSV, but the antibodies do not afford lifelong protection. Subsequent reinfections are usually milder than initial infections.

Can RSV infection be lethal?
There is no medication available to treat severe RSV. RSV is an important cause of mortality in young children and is estimated to be second only to malaria as a source of infant mortality worldwide. RSV also is a significant cause of mortality among older people.

What are risk factors for developing severe RSV disease?
Babies born during or just before RSV season (late fall and winter) are at higher risk of severe RSV infection. Infection

rates peak in infants who are 2 months old because maternal antibodies wane and these infants have not developed their own. Having older siblings is a risk factor because they are more likely to transmit an infection. People older than age 60 years are also at higher risk for severe disease, as are people who are immunocompromised and those with cardiovascular and pulmonary disease.

Is nirsevimab a vaccine?

Nirsevimab is a monoclonal antibody product that is a passive immunization. Although not technically a "vaccine" in a traditional sense (active immunization), it is being used in a manner similar to routine childhood vaccines and may be referred to as a vaccine by some entities. Nirsevimab confers long-lasting protection from RSV, with protection expected to last at least 5 months (about the length of a typical RSV season). Nirsevimab is part of the Vaccines for Children program.

How long does the RSV protection conferred by nirsevimab last?

Protection is expected to last at least 5 months, about the length of an RSV season, and is expected to reduce the risk of severe RSV disease by approximately 80%.

Can my baby receive nirsevimab if I received RSV vaccine during my pregnancy?

The CDC recommends that nirsevimab be given to infants younger than 8 months of age born during or entering the RSV season if their mother did not receive RSV vaccine, the mother's vaccination status is unknown, or the infant is born less than 14 days after the mother's vaccination.

DENGUE

Did you know that:

- The word "dengue" is derived from the Swahili phrase *Kadinga pepo*, meaning "cramp-like seizure."
- Almost half of the world's population, approximately 4 billion people, live in areas with a risk of dengue.
- It is estimated that 100 to 400 million dengue infections occur each year.
- Dengue viruses are highly mobile and are transported all over the world by infected travelers.

Dengue has been recognized for over 3 centuries. The first clinically recognized dengue epidemics occurred almost simultaneously in Asia, Africa, and North America in the 1780s. Dengue is a vector-borne infectious disease caused by four dengue viral serotypes (DENV-1, DENV-2, DENV-3, and DENV-4) that are part of the genus *Flavivirus*. Infection with one of the serotypes is not cross-protective. The viruses are transmitted by *Aedes aegypti* and *Aedes albopictus* mosquitos. The disease is endemic in Africa, the Americas, and areas of the Middle East, Asia, and the Western Pacific. Since 1980, the frequency of dengue infections and its more severe complications (dengue hemorrhagic fever and dengue shock syndrome) has been dramatically increasing.

Infection with dengue viruses produces a range of clinical illness, from a nonspecific viral syndrome to severe and fatal hemorrhagic disease. Dengue may occur in persons of all ages, with the highest rates in adolescents and young adults. In endemic areas, most of the deaths from dengue infection occur in children younger than 15 years of age. It is most likely to cause severe disease in infants, pregnant women, and patient with chronic diseases (e.g., asthma, diabetes mellitus, and sickle cell anemia). If a person has a medical history of dengue fever and becomes infected again, there is a significantly increased risk of developing serious and life-threatening dengue hemorrhagic fever (severe shock, respiratory distress, severe bleeding, multiorgan dysfunction, impaired consciousness, and neurologic disease including acute meningoencephalitis).

Transmission

The viruses are transmitted through bites from *A. aegypti* and *A. albopictus* mosquitos.

Incubation Period

The incubation period for dengue virus replication in mosquitoes is 8 to 12 days, with the mosquitoes remaining infectious for the remainder of their life cycle. In humans, the incubation period is 3 to 14 days before symptom onset. Infected people, both asymptomatic and symptomatic, can transmit dengue virus to mosquitoes 1 or 2 days before symptoms develop and throughout the approximately 7-day viremic period.

Treatment

There is no specific effective antiviral therapy for dengue infection. Treatment is supportive, with particular attention to fluid management.

Prevention

Dengue vaccine (Dengvaxia) is a recombinant, live, attenuated chimeric tetravalent vaccine built on a yellow fever 17D backbone. It is administered as a 3-dose series at 0, 6, and 12 months only to persons who have laboratory evidence of a previous dengue infection. Vaccine efficacy ranges from 67% to 82% against the four different serotypes in the vaccine in the prevention of severe dengue disease and hospitalization. Vaccine may be administered to persons 9 to 45 years of age who are living in dengue endemic areas and have laboratory confirmation of a previous dengue infection. Prior natural infection is important because dengue vaccination is associated with an increased risk for severe dengue in those who have their initial dengue infection after vaccination. In the United States, dengue vaccine is only for use in persons living in U.S. territories and freely associated states where dengue is endemic, including Puerto Rico, American Samoa, U.S. Virgin Islands, Federated States of Micronesia, Republic of Marshall Islands, and the Republic of Palau.

Duration of Immunity

At least 6 years after the last dose of vaccine

Contraindications and Precautions

Contraindications
1. A person who has immunodeficiency or immunosuppression due to underlying disease or therapy, including symptomatic HIV infection of CD4$^+$ T-lymphocyte count of <200/uL

2. A person who lacks laboratory evidence of previous dengue infection
3. A person who has ever had a severe allergic reaction (e.g., anaphylaxis) after a previous dose of this vaccine
4. A person who has a severe allergy to any vaccine component

Precautions
1. Breastfeeding
2. Pregnancy
3. People with HIV
4. Persons with moderate or severe acute illness with or without fever

Frequently Asked Questions

If I am traveling to visit family who live in a dengue endemic area but I do not live there, can I get dengue vaccine?
In the United States, dengue vaccine is only for use in persons living in U.S. territories and freely associated states where dengue is endemic, including Puerto Rico, American Samoa, U.S. Virgin Islands, Federated States of Micronesia, Republic of Marshall Islands, and the Republic of Palau. The person must have laboratory evidence of a previous dengue infection before they can receive the vaccine. The dengue vaccine is not recommended for other travelers who do not reside in these areas.

If you get dengue fever once, can you get it again?
Yes. There are four major serotypes of dengue viruses (DENV-1, DENV-2, DENV-3, and DENV-4). Having dengue fever with one type of dengue virus will not protect you from the other three types.

How can you prevent getting dengue fever again?
1. When traveling to areas that have dengue fever, try to avoid exposure to mosquitoes and use insect repellent if going to areas with a lot of mosquitoes. *Aedes* mosquitoes are usually most active in the early morning hours after daybreak, in the late afternoon before dark, and any time during the day when indoors or in shady areas.
2. Make sure screens on windows and doorways do not have holes.
3. Mosquito netting over beds may be helpful if you tend to take naps during the early morning and evening hours or during the day when these mosquitoes are active.
4. If you reside in a dengue endemic area, get vaccinated with dengue vaccine.

REFERENCE

Paz-Bailey G, Adams L, Wong JM, et al. Dengue vaccine: Recommendations of the Advisory Committee on Immunization Practices, United States, 2021. *MMWR Recomm Rep.* 2021;70(No. RR-6):1–16.

MPOX

Did you know that:

- The name monkeypox (mpox) originates from the discovery of the virus during an outbreak among monkeys in a Danish laboratory in 1958.
- The first documented human case of mpox was identified in a 9-month-old infant in the Democratic Republic of the Congo (DRC) in 1970.

- In countries with a history of mpox, the largest numbers of cases have been reported in Nigeria, the DRC, and Ghana.
- In 2003, 47 cases of mpox were reported in six Midwestern U.S. states. All those cases of infection occurred following contact with pet prairie dogs. The pets were infected after being housed near imported small mammals from Ghana. This was the first time that human mpox was reported outside of Africa.
- The 2022 mpox epidemic has infected more than 90,000 persons worldwide in 110 locations that had not historically reported disease. Through 2023, more than 30,000 cases and 55 deaths have been reported.

Mpox virus is a DNA virus in the *Orthopoxvirus* genus, which also includes viruses such as vaccinia, cowpox, and variola. The principal symptoms of mpox infection are fever, chills, and malaise followed by the development of a centrifugal rash involving the palms of the hands and soles of the feet. Fever can last for up to 1 week, and the rash evolves from maculopapular to vesicular to pustular to crusting over a period of 2 to 4 weeks. Unlike smallpox, typical mpox infections are usually characterized by lymphadenopathy. In the recent global outbreak, mpox has often presented without fever or rash, and with only one to a few skin lesions. Often, these lesions have been present on the genitalia, oral mucosa, or rectal mucosa, consistent with the points of intimate contact.

Transmission

Although mpox was originally described in monkeys in 1958, rodents are likely to be the natural reservoir of this virus, and primates—including humans—are incidental hosts. The major risk for infection currently is among men who have sex with men; transmission appears to be limited to skin-to-skin, oral, and rectal and perianal intimate contact, and possibly through semen.

Incubation Period

The incubation period of mpox infection ranges from 7 to 21 days, with shorter incubation periods occurring with more invasive exposure.

Prevention

In the 1960s, investigators reported that monkeys could be immunized against mpox by smallpox vaccination. A later analysis of human mpox cases in Central Africa calculated that previous smallpox vaccination (defined by the presence of vaccination scar) conferred 85% protection against mpox disease. The cessation of the smallpox vaccination program in 1980 may have contributed to the current mpox outbreak by decreasing herd immunity.

Smallpox and mpox vaccines can be used in two situations: pre-exposure to prevent infection and disease or post-exposure to ameliorate infection and disease.

Pre-exposure Vaccination
Pre-exposure vaccination is warranted to protect those at the highest risk, especially men who have sex with men with multiple sexual partners.

Post-exposure Vaccination
Ideally, post-exposure vaccination is administered within 4 days of exposure to prevent infection, but it can be used up to 14 days after exposure to decrease the severity of disease.

Currently in the United States, there are two licensed smallpox vaccines: ACAM2000 and JYNNEOS. ACAM2000 is licensed to prevent smallpox and made available for use against mpox under an Expanded Access Investigational New Drug protocol. JYNNEOS is approved for the prevention of both smallpox and mpox. Another vaccinia virus vaccine, LC16m18, is available in Japan.

- ACAM2000
  Second-generation replication-competent live vaccinia virus. A single dose administered via bifurcated needle
- LC16m18
  Third-generation, attenuated, minimally replication-competent vaccinia virus. A single dose administered via bifurcated needle
- JYNNEOS
  Third-generation, replication-deficient modified live, attenuated vaccinia Ankara. Two doses, 28 days apart, administered subcutaneously (0.5 mL) or intradermal (0.1 mL)

JYNNEOS is a third-generation vaccine based on the non-replicating modified live, attenuated vaccinia virus Ankara (MVA) strain with deletion of approximately 10% of its genome. With 2 doses, immunogenicity is similar to that seen with ACAM2000, but with fewer adverse events. During the current outbreak, JYNNEOS is the main vaccine being used in the United States. Limited data on performance of JYNNEOS vaccine in the current outbreak are available. The CDC has reported that mpox incidence was 14-fold higher among unvaccinated males compared with those who had received a first vaccine dose at least 14 days earlier.

Duration of Immunity

Unknown at this time

Adverse Events

MVA-based vaccines do not elicit the characteristic "take" seen with earlier smallpox vaccines. Earlier smallpox vaccines typically resulted in a localized vaccinia infection at the inoculation site—a skin lesion that progressed from papule to vesicle to pustule to scab over 2 or 3 weeks. MVA-based vaccines are associated with many of the same common, mild side effects, including pain at the site of injection (85% of recipients); redness, swelling, itching, and induration at the site of injection (40–60%); fatigue, muscle pain, and headaches (20–40%); nausea (17%); and chills (10%). Only approximately 2% of recipients report fever. Similarly, cardiac events were reported in about 2% of recipients, but myopericarditis was not seen.

Contraindications and Precautions to Mpox Vaccines

Contraindications

Persons who experienced a severe allergic reaction following a previous dose of JYNNEOS or following exposure to any component of JYNNEOS may be at increased risk for severe allergic reactions after JYNNEOS. The risk for a severe allergic reaction should be weighed against the risk for disease due to smallpox or mpox.

Precautions
1. Immunocompromised persons, including those receiving immunosuppressive therapy, may have a diminished immune response to JYNNEOS.

2. Vaccination with JYNNEOS may not protect all recipients.
3. Developmental toxicity studies conducted in female rats and rabbits demonstrated no evidence of harm to the fetus, but there are insufficient human data to inform vaccine-associated risks in pregnancy.
4. No information is available on the clinical use of mpox vaccine during breastfeeding.

Frequently Asked Questions

After completion of the primary vaccine series, will additional booster doses be necessary?
No additional booster doses of mpox vaccine are recommended at this time.

How long is mpox contagious?
Mpox can spread from the time symptoms start until the rash has fully healed and a fresh layer of skin has formed, which usually takes 2 to 4 weeks.

Can mpox be transmitted to pets?
Mpox can spread to animals, so staying away from pets and other animals is recommended.

Are mpox vaccines safe?
Both JYNNEOS and ACAM2000 have FDA approval for use against poxviruses. They were cleared for use after extensive testing in people. JYNNEOS has been associated with few possible complications. It can be given even to people with weakened immunity. ACAM2000 has been associated with a risk of myocarditis and pericarditis. Risk is higher for those who have

never had a smallpox vaccine, such as most people younger than age 60 years.

The CDC recommends that ACAM2000 should not be given to people who

- have severely weakened immunity;
- are living with HIV;
- have skin conditions such as eczema or psoriasis;
- have heart disease;
- have eye disease treated with topical steroids;
- are pregnant; and
- are younger than age 12 months

Who should get the mpox vaccine?
1. Anyone who has had close contact with someone diagnosed with mpox (e.g., household members with close physical contact or intimate partners)
2. Gay, bisexual, and other men who have sex with men and/or transgender persons who are sexually active
3. Lab workers who do mpox tests
4. Health care workers who have been exposed to mpox without personal protective equipment

Should children be vaccinated against mpox?
Children may be eligible for vaccination if they have had close personal contact with someone who has or may have mpox.

What should be done if the second dose is delayed?
The second dose may be given up to 7 days later than the minimum interval of 28 days (i.e., up to 35 days after the first dose).

Does previous receipt of smallpox vaccine provide protection against mpox?
Prior receipt of smallpox vaccine appears to provide some protection against mpox. The United States stopped routine smallpox vaccination in 1972.

Can you get mpox more than once?
Reinfection has been reported. Less severe mpox disease has been reported both in people with previous infection and in people who were vaccinated.

PART IV

TRAVEL VACCINES

YELLOW FEVER VACCINE

Did you know that:

- The earliest recorded record of yellow fever comes from a Mayan manuscript discovered in the Yucatan from 1648.
- Yellow fever was a major problem in the 18th century in colonial settlements in the Americas and West Africa. The disease was repeatedly introduced into seaports in the United States via sailing vessels infested with *Aedes aegypti* mosquitos that sustained transmission among the passengers and crew.
- In 1793, an outbreak of yellow fever in Philadelphia, which at the time was the federal capital of the United States, killed 10% of the population.
- The sweat of a person with yellow fever smells like a butcher's shop.

Yellow fever (YF) is transmitted in forested areas of sub-Saharan Africa and South America but may spread to urban areas and in dry locations where stored water provides breeding sites. Figure

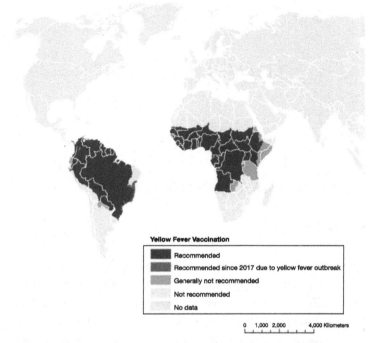

Figure 8 Areas of the world where yellow fever is endemic. *Source: Data from the Centers for Disease Control and Prevention, 2020, https://rb.gy/hoeeii.*

8 shows the areas of the world where YF is endemic. YF illness ranges in severity from a self-limited, febrile illness to hemorrhagic fever that is fatal in 50% of cases. Up to 50% of infections are asymptomatic. After an incubation period of 3 to 6 days, fever, headache, and myalgias begin abruptly, accompanied by conjunctival injection, facial flushing, relative bradycardia, and leukopenia. In most cases, these symptoms resolve with no further complications. In severe cases, after a short period of resolution, the symptoms return with high fever, headache, back pain, nausea, vomiting, abdominal pain, and somnolence. This is followed by

severe weakness; icteric hepatitis; and prominent gastrointestinal bleeding, hematemesis, epistaxis, gum bleeding, and petechial and purpuric hemorrhages. Ultimately, hypotension, shock, and metabolic acidosis develop, accompanied by myocardial dysfunction, arrhythmias, azotemia, confusion, seizures, and coma. Death may occur within 7 to 10 days. A traveler's risk for acquiring YF is determined by various factors, including immunization status, location of travel, season of year, duration of exposure, occupational and recreational activities while traveling, and local rate of virus transmission at the time of travel. From 1970 through 2015, a total of 11 cases of YF were reported in unvaccinated travelers from the United States and Europe who traveled to West Africa (6 cases) or South America (5 cases). Eight (73%) of these 11 travelers died. The risk of acquiring YF is difficult to predict because of variations in ecologic determinants of virus transmission. For a 2-week stay, the estimated risks for illness and death due to YF for an unvaccinated traveler visiting an endemic area in West Africa and South America are as follows:

- West Africa: 50 per 100,000 and 10 per 100,000, respectively
- South America: 5 per 100,000 and 1 per 100,000, respectively

Transmission

Yellow fever is transmitted by *A. aegypti* mosquitoes. The mosquitoes are infected after feeding on viremic humans and then spread the infection during subsequent feedings.

Incubation Period

3 to 6 days after bite from infected mosquito

Treatment

No antiviral therapy is available. Treatment is supportive care.

Prevention

Pre-exposure Prophylaxis
Yellow fever vaccine—live, attenuated 17D vaccine that is administered subcutaneously as single dose. Vaccine should be administered at least 10 days prior to travel. Compulsory vaccine is required by certain countries for entry and can only be administered by certified travel clinics. Vaccine may be administered with other live vaccines. If not given at the same time, other live vaccines should be given 3 weeks later.

Duration of Immunity

Probably lifelong after 1 dose; however, a booster dose is recommended every 10 years if a person resides or frequently travels to an endemic area or if the foreign country requires it for entry.

Contraindications and Precautions to Yellow Fever Vaccine

Contraindications

1. Immunocompromised host, including due to immunosuppressive and immunomodulatory therapies
2. Anaphylactic reaction to eggs/egg products or prior dose of vaccine and any of its components
3. Age younger than 6 months, except during epidemics

Precautions
1. Infants between 6 and 8 months of age and persons 60 years of age or older due to a very small increased risk of post-vaccination encephalitis (1 person in 125,000).
2. Pregnancy—not recommended unless travel to a high-risk endemic area cannot be avoided or postponed. In areas where YF is endemic, or during outbreaks, the benefits of YF vaccination are likely to far outweigh the risk of potential transmission of vaccine virus to the fetus or infant. Pregnant women and nursing mothers should be counseled on the potential benefits and risks of vaccination so that they may make an informed decision about vaccination.
3. Breastfeeding—lactating women should be advised that the benefits of breastfeeding far outweigh alternatives. Vaccination is recommended, if indicated, for breastfeeding women traveling to endemic areas when such travel cannot be avoided or postponed or during epidemics.

Frequently Asked Questions

Does a patient need to avoid contact with immunocompromised family members after receiving the YF vaccine?
No. There is no evidence that people who receive YF vaccine shed the vaccine virus. Therefore, there is no need to avoid contact with persons who have weak immune systems.

How long should a woman wait to conceive after receiving a YF vaccination?
YF vaccination has not been known to cause any birth defects when given to pregnant women and has been given to many pregnant women without any apparent adverse effects on the

fetus. However, because YF vaccine is a live virus vaccine, it poses a theoretical risk. Although a 2-week delay between YF vaccination and conception is probably adequate, a 1-month delay has been advocated as a more conservative approach. If a woman is inadvertently or of necessity vaccinated during pregnancy, she is unlikely to have any problems from the vaccine and her baby is very likely to be born healthy.

Why is YF vaccine not recommended to be given to adults aged 60 years or older even if they are traveling to an endemic area of the world?
People aged 60 years or older may be at increased risk for serious adverse events (serious disease or, very rarely, death) following vaccination compared with younger persons. This is particularly true if they are receiving their first YF vaccination. Travelers aged 60 years or older should discuss with their health care provider the risks and benefits of the vaccine given their travel plans. In addition to considering the vaccine, travelers to endemic areas should protect themselves from YF and other vector-borne diseases. Preventive measures include wearing clothes with long sleeves and long pants and using an effective insect repellent such as those with DEET, picaridin, IR3535, or oil of lemon eucalyptus.

TYPHOID FEVER VACCINE

Did you know that:

- Mary Mallon (aka "Typhoid Mary") immigrated from a small village in Northern Ireland in 1883 and served as a cook to wealthy families in New York City. She was

responsible for at least two separate typhoid fever outbreaks resulting in infection of 51 persons and 3 deaths. It is presumed that her poor hand hygiene was what allowed her to spread disease so effectively.
- Typhoid Mary spent a total of 26 years in forced isolation to prevent the spread of the disease. She died in 1938 while still in isolation.
- Typhoid Mary was the first person in the United States identified as an asymptomatic carrier of the typhoid fever organism.
- Wolfgang Amadeus Mozart suffered from smallpox and a bout of typhoid fever during his lifetime.
- The sweat of a person with typhoid fever smells like freshly baked bread.

Typhoid fever is a global health problem, with an estimated 21 million cases worldwide and 200,000 deaths each year. The disease is very common in developing countries, especially in the Indian subcontinent (India and Pakistan), Southeast Asia, South and Central America, and Africa. It is caused by several typhoidal *Salmonella* species, including *S. typhi*, *S. enterica* subtype Enteritidis, and *S. paratyphi*. The onset of disease is gradual, with symptoms ranging from mild to severe. The most common manifestations are high fever, headache, malaise, anorexia, lethargy, abdominal tenderness, hepatosplenomegaly, diarrhea or constipation, rose-colored spots on the trunk or abdomen, and changes in mental status. Persons with typhoid fever may excrete *Salmonella* organisms in their stools for months after having typhoid fever. This serves as a source of infection to their contacts. Complications may occur in up to 15% of patients. The most common complications include gastrointestinal bleeding, intestinal perforation, hepatitis, and encephalopathy. Even after receiving appropriate therapy, 5% to 10% of patients will relapse approximately 1 to 3 weeks after recovering from the initial illness, and it is often milder than the initial illness. A chronic carrier state, in which stool or urine cultures for *S. typhi* remain positive for more than 1 year, occurs in up to 5% of infected people.

Transmission

Acquisition of infection occurs by ingestion of fecally contaminated food or water (e.g., through handling by a person who is shedding *S. typhi* or if sewage contaminates the water used for drinking or washing food). Therefore, typhoid fever is more common in areas of the world where proper handwashing is less frequent and water is likely to be contaminated with sewage.

Incubation Period

Incubation period is on average 8 to 14 days, but it ranges from 3 to 60 days or more.

Treatment

Third-generation cephalosporins, azithromycin, and fluoroquinolones are first-line antibiotics. Response to antibiotic therapy is slow, and fever may persist for many days and even weeks after the patient's blood culture has cleared.

Prevention

Pre-exposure Prophylaxis
Typhoid fever vaccine dosage and delivery are summarized in Table 17.

Table 17 TYPHOID FEVER VACCINES

Vaccine Name	Type of Vaccine	How Given	Number of Doses Necessary	Time Between Doses	Time Immunization Should Be Completed by (Before Possible Exposure)	Minimum Age for Vaccination	Booster Needed Every...
Ty21a (Vivotif Berna, Swiss Serum and Vaccine Institute)	Live, attenuated, oral	PO—by mouth	4	2 days	1 week	6 years	5 years
ViCPS (Typhim Vi, Pasteur Merieux)	Inactivated	IM—injection	1	N/A	2 weeks	2 years	2 years

N/A, not applicable.

Contraindications and Precautions to Typhoid Fever Vaccine

Contraindications
1. Persons with history of anaphylaxis after previous administration of the vaccine and in persons with suspected or proven hypersensitivity to any component of the vaccine
2. For oral live, attenuated vaccine
    i. Pregnancy
    ii. Individuals with an acute gastrointestinal condition or inflammatory bowel disease
    iii. Persons with known or suspected immunocompromising condition

Precautions
1. Persons with severe acute illness with or without fever
2. For oral live, attenuated vaccine
    i. Persons who are taking antibiotics or certain antimalarials that may kill the organism in the vaccine

Frequently Asked Questions

How long can an infected person carry the typhoid fever bacteria?
The duration of the carrier stage varies from days to years. Only approximately 3% of patients go on to become lifelong carriers, and this tends to occur more often in adults than in children.

One of my relatives returned from a trip to Pakistan and has typhoid fever. Should my relative be kept away from other family members when they return home?

Only people with active diarrhea who are unable to control their bowels (e.g., infants, certain disabled individuals, and persons with copious diarrhea) should be isolated. Most infected people may return to work or school when they have been appropriately treated with antibiotics, provided they carefully wash their hands after using the toilet. Children in day care should obtain approval from the Department of Public Health before returning to their routine activities. Food handlers and those who provide patient care *may not* return to work until three consecutive negative stool specimens are obtained.

JAPANESE ENCEPHALITIS VACCINE

Did you know that:

- Mosquito larvae infected with the Japanese encephalitis virus are found in flooded rice fields, marshes, and small stable collections of water around cultivated fields. Pigs and certain species of wild birds amplify the virus in their bloodstreams when infected, so areas where these animals are prevalent are areas of highest risk. Habitats supporting the transmission cycle of Japanese encephalitis virus are principally in rural, pig farming, and rice patty locations. Traveling and living "off the grid" in these locations place one at high risk for contracting this disease.
- Seizures occur in more than 75% of pediatric patients with the disease but much less frequently in adults.
- Japanese encephalitis is the leading cause of vaccine-preventable encephalitis in Asia and the western Pacific.

Japanese encephalitis (JE) virus is a flavivirus that is an arthropod-borne infection. It is transmitted in Asia over an area spanning one-third of the world's circumference, from Pakistan at the westernmost edge to far eastern Russia. The disease is endemic and epidemic in Southeast Asia, China, and the Asian subcontinent, including Indonesian and the Philippines (see Figure 9 for endemic areas). Most infections with JE virus are asymptomatic. In countries where disease is endemic, infections acquired naturally at an early age result in immunity in more than 80% of young adults. Symptomatic infections occur primarily in children between ages 2 and 10 years, with a higher incidence in males. Travelers of *all* ages without naturally acquired protective antibodies are at risk for acquisition of the illness. Infection is symptomatic in less than 1% of cases of JE, but the illness usually presents as a severe encephalitis, leading frequently to coma and to a fatal outcome in 25% of cases.

The earliest symptoms are lethargy, fever, headache, abdominal pain, nausea, and vomiting. Lethargy increases over several days associated with agitated delirium, unsteadiness, and abnormal motor movements, advancing to progressive somnolence and coma. Multiple seizures and status epilepticus are associated with a poor outcome. Neurologic abnormalities persist in up to one-third of patients. A large proportion of recovered children (up to 75%) exhibit behavioral and psychological abnormalities. Illness acquired in the first and second trimesters of pregnancy may precipitate abortion.

Incubation

Incubation period is 5 to 15 days after being bitten by an infected mosquito.

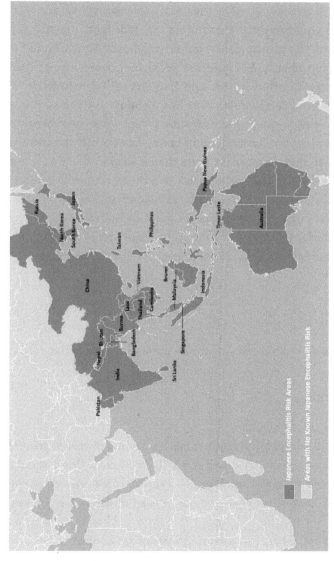

Figure 9 Map of countries in Asia and the western Pacific in which Japanese encephalitis virus has been identified.

Transmission

The virus is transmitted by the *Culex tritaeniorhynchus* and related ground-pool-breeding mosquitoes to pigs and aquatic birds, which are the principal viral amplifying hosts. Viremic adult pigs are asymptomatic, but infected pregnant sows abort or deliver stillbirths. Infected horses and humans are symptomatic. Rice paddies provide favorable breeding habitats for vector mosquitoes; therefore, the risk of infection is highest in rural areas with rice growing, pig farming, and horses, especially if the traveler is staying in this this area for more than 3 weeks.

Travelers at the highest risk are those who will be staying in rural rice-growing and pig-farming endemic areas for at least 3 weeks; engaging in extensive outdoor activities (e.g., camping, hiking, fishing, and biking) in rural areas; and staying in accommodations that lack window screens, air-conditioning, or bed nets.

Treatment

There is no specific therapy for JE outside of supportive care.

Prevention

Pre-exposure Prophylaxis
Japanese encephalitis vaccine: Ixaro is an inactivated vaccine that is a 2-dose series with doses given 28 days apart. Doses should be completed at least 1 week prior to travel. It is licensed for use in persons 2 months of age or older. It is administered as follows:

- A 0.5 mL IM dose to persons 3 years of age or older
- A 0.25 mL IM dose to persons 2 months through 2 years of age

Booster Dose
Recommended for persons 17 years of age or older if continued exposure anticipated and more than 1 year has elapsed since completion of the primary 2-dose series.

Contraindications and Precautions to Japanese Encephalitis Vaccine

Contraindications
1. Severe allergic reaction (e.g., anaphylaxis) to a previous dose of vaccine or any vaccine component

Precautions
1. Moderate or severe acute illness with or without fever
2. Pregnancy—theoretical risk to the fetus; however, no deleterious effects have been demonstrated from JE vaccine administration during pregnancy, and the risk of adverse fetal effects from an inactivated vaccine is extremely low

Duration of Protection

Unknown

Frequently Asked Questions

Can a person get infected through close contact with an infected person?
No. The JE virus has not been shown to be transmitted from person to person.

Can a person contract JE through eating pork that comes from an endemic area?

No. Once the pig is slaughtered, the JE virus will not survive in the pork meat. The JE virus can only survive in living cells. Any virus will be killed by cooking, roasting, or boiling the meat at a temperature of more than 60°C, and the digestive enzymes and acid in people's stomachs will also kill the virus.

RABIES VACCINE

Did you know that:

- The earliest reported description of rabies is before 2300 BC in the Mesopotamian Laws of Eshnunna.
- Quote from Lewis Thomas in *The Lives of a Cell*, 1974: "I have seen agony in death only once, in a patient with rabies: He remained acutely aware of every stage in the process of his own disintegration over a twenty four-hour period, right up to his final moment."
- Indoor-only pets can get rabies when they come into contact with rabid animals that enter the home. Bats—the most common rabid animal in the United States—enter homes and can bite or scratch pets.

Rabies is an acute illness with rapidly progressive central nervous system manifestations, including anxiety, radicular pain, dysesthesia or pruritus, hydrophobia, and dysautonomia or paralysis. Illness almost invariably progresses to death. The disease has three sequential stages: (1) the prodromal stage, which lasts for 2 to 10 days and is characterized by fever, headache, malaise, fatigue, anorexia, anxiety, agitation, irritability, insomnia, depression, and pain, pruritus, or paresthesia at the site of the bite; (2) the acute neurologic state, which lasts 2 to 12 days and is characterized by hyperactivity, disorientation, hallucinations, bizarre behavior, aggressiveness, seizures, paralysis, aerophobia, hyperventilation, and cholinergic manifestations, including hypersalivation, lacrimation, mydriasis, and hyperpyrexia, with paralysis occurring in 20% of cases; and (3) at the end of the neurologic stage, the patient may become comatose. Death from cardiorespiratory arrest usually occurs within 7 days, although with supportive care, coma may last for months. Each year, there are an estimated 59,000 human rabies cases worldwide, with only 1 to 3 cases occurring in the United States. Disease is almost 100% fatal.

Transmission

The virus is present in the saliva of a number of different animals and is transmitted by bites or by contamination of mucosa or skin lesions by saliva or other potentially infectious material. In the United States, bats, raccoons, skunks, foxes, wolves, coyotes, and bobcats are the most important sources of infection for humans and domestic animals. Worldwide, most human cases of rabies result from dog or cat bites. Transmission also has occurred by transplantation of organs, corneas, and other tissues from patients dying of undiagnosed rabies.

Incubation Period

The incubation period is 1 to 3 months, but it ranges from days to years.

Treatment

There is no specific treatment.

Prevention

Post-exposure

a. Post-exposure prophylaxis is recommended for all persons bitten by wild mammalian carnivores or bats or by domestic animals that are suspected to be rabid. It is also recommended for people who report an open wound, scratch, or mucous membrane that has been contaminated with saliva or other potentially infectious material from a rabid animal.

b. The injury inflicted by a bat bite or scratch may be small and not readily evident, or the circumstances of contact with a bat may preclude accurate recall (e.g., a bat in a room of a deeply sleeping or medicated person, or an unattended child, especially an infant or toddler who cannot reliably communicate about a potential bite). Therefore, post-exposure prophylaxis may be indicated in situations in which a bat physically is present in the same room if a bite or mucous membrane exposure cannot reliably be excluded, unless prompt testing of the bat has excluded rabies virus infection. **Prophylaxis should be initiated as soon as possible after bites by known or suspected rabid animals.**

c. The immediate objective of post-exposure prophylaxis is to prevent virus from entering neural tissue. Prompt and thorough local treatment of all lesions is essential because virus may remain localized to the area of the bite for a variable time. All wounds should be flushed thoroughly and cleaned with soap and water. **After wound care is completed, concurrent use of passive and active prophylaxis is optimal.** The exception is in persons who previously have received complete vaccination regimens with a cell culture vaccine or people who have been vaccinated with other types of rabies vaccines and have previously had a documented rabies virus-neutralizing antibody titer; these people should receive only vaccine.

d. Prophylaxis should begin as soon as possible after exposure, **ideally within 24 hours.** However, a delay of several days or more may not compromise effectiveness, and **prophylaxis should be initiated if reasonably indicated, regardless of the interval between exposure and initiation of therapy.**

Passive prophylaxis—rabies immune globulin (RIG)—in the United States, only human RIG is available. The dosing is 20 IU/kg—wound site should be infiltrated with as much of the RIG as possible and any remaining volume should be administered intramuscularly. This should be used concomitantly with the first dose of vaccine to bridge the time between possible infection and antibody production induced by the vaccine.

Active prophylaxis—human diploid cell vaccine (Imovax) and purified chicken embryo cell vaccine (RabAvert) are available for use in the United States.

a. For a previously unvaccinated immunocompetent person, a 1.0 mL dose of vaccine is given IM in the deltoid area (the anterolateral aspect of the thigh is also acceptable for children) on the first day of post-exposure prophylaxis (day 0), and repeated doses are given on days 3, 7, and 14 after the first dose for a total of 4 doses, with 1 dose of RIG given on day 0.

b. For a person with altered immunocompetence, post-exposure prophylaxis should include a 5-dose vaccination regimen (i.e., 1 dose of vaccine on days 0, 3, 7, 14, and 28), with 1 dose of RIG on day 0.

Pre-exposure
  a. Pre-exposure prophylaxis is recommended for people in high-risk groups, including veterinarians, animal handlers, certain laboratory workers, and people moving or traveling to areas where canine rabies is common. Others, such as spelunkers (cavers) or animal rehabilitators, who may have frequent exposures to bats and other wildlife, should also be considered for pre-exposure prophylaxis.
  b. The pre-exposure prophylaxis vaccine schedule is a 2-dose series given as a 1.0 mL IM injection on days 0 and 7.

Duration of Protection

Serum antibodies usually persist for 3 years or longer after the primary series is administered intramuscularly.

Contraindications and Precautions for Rabies Vaccine

Contraindications
  1. In the situation of exposure to rabies, there are no contraindications to vaccination or use of human RIG.

Precautions
  1. Severe allergic reaction (e.g., anaphylaxis) to a previous dose of vaccine or any vaccine component
  2. Immunosuppression—immunosuppressive agents should not be administered during post-exposure prophylaxis unless absolutely essential. If possible, pre-exposure prophylaxis should be postponed until immunocompromising conditions are resolved. When an immunosuppressed

person is given pre- or post-exposure prophylaxis, antibody titers should be checked.
3. Patients with selective IgA deficiency may be at increased risk for anaphylactic reactions to human RIG because it may contain trace amounts of IgA.

Frequently Asked Questions

My granddaughter just received two hamsters for her birthday. Can these small rodents transmit rabies to humans?
Rabies in small rodents (e.g., squirrels, hamsters, guinea pigs, gerbils, chipmunks, rats, and mice) and lagomorphs such as rabbits, pikas, and hares is very rare, and these animals do not pose a rabies infection risk.

Is it possible to develop rabies from the rabies vaccine?
No. All rabies vaccines used in humans are inactivated and therefore it is not possible for the vaccine to cause disease.

Is a human infected with rabies able to transmit the disease to other humans?
Person-to-person transmission has never been documented; however, precautions should be taken to prevent exposure to the saliva of a diseased person. Very rarely, rabies has been transmitted from infected tissue that was transplanted into an uninfected person.

What animal worldwide is the major source of rabies?
Dogs are the main source of human rabies deaths, contributing up to 99% of all rabies transmissions to humans.

CHOLERA VACCINE

Did you know that:

- Reports of cholera-like disease have been found as early as 1000 AD.
- Cholera has the distinction of being among the most rapidly fatal infectious diseases of humans, with the ability to cause death within 6 to 12 hours of onset of clinical symptoms.
- Prior to the development of effective rehydration therapy with intravenous and oral fluids, cholera epidemics were associated with case-fatality rates that exceeded 60% and led to tens of thousands of deaths.
- The diarrhea of cholera is described as "rice-water stool." The stools are watery and often contain flecks of whitish material (mucus and some gastrointestinal lining cells) that are approximately the size of pieces of rice, and the stools smell "fishy."
- The volume of diarrhea can be enormous, with as much as 250 cc/kg or approximately 10 to 18 liters of diarrhea fluid lost over a 24-hour period.

Cholera is an acute, rapidly dehydrating, watery, painless diarrheal disease caused by infection with toxogenic strains of the bacterium *Vibrio cholerae* serogroups O1 and O139. Serogroup O1 is the most common. The World Health Organization (WHO) estimates that approximately 3 to 5 million people are infected worldwide each year, with approximately 100,000 deaths per year. Figure 10 shows the areas of the world where cholera outbreaks continue to be a problem. Cholera is now endemic in more than 50 countries

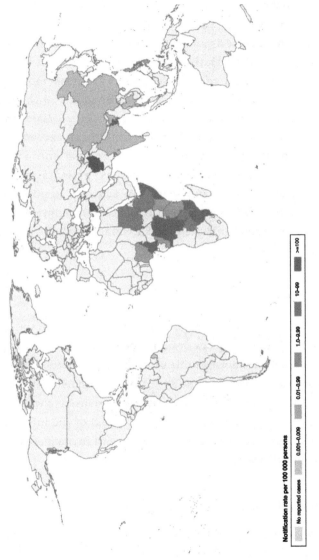

Figure 10 Areas of the world where cholera outbreaks continue. *Source: European Centre for Disease Prevention and Control.*

and can appear in explosive epidemics. Since the early 1800s, there have been seven cholera pandemics. The current pandemic began in 1961 and is caused by *V. cholerae* O1 El Tor.

Cholera manifests as an acute, severe watery, painless diarrhea that can lead to death from dehydration within hours of onset. The spectrum of disease ranges from asymptomatic intestinal colonization (observed in individuals with preexisting immunity) to mild, moderate, and severe diarrhea. In severe diarrhea, the volume of watery stool can exceed 1 liter per hour. Vomiting is common, however, and patients are usually afebrile. As the dehydration worsens, patients may also experience muscle pain and spasm. In addition to potentially life-threatening dehydration and hypovolemia, common complications of cholera include hypokalemia, metabolic acidosis, and hypoglycemia.

Transmission

Transmission occurs through the consumption of contaminated water or food (especially raw or undercooked shellfish, raw or partially dried fish, or moist grains or vegetables stored at ambient temperature) and is often the result of a combined contamination. For example, contaminated water is often used to wash fresh food, thereby contaminating the food. Spread of the infection is by the fecal–oral route and is associated with inadequate sanitation and unsafe water.

Incubation Period

The incubation period is 1 to 3 days, with a range of a few hours to 5 days.

Treatment

a. The cornerstone of management is appropriate rehydration therapy. Rehydration therapy should be based on WHO standards, with the goal of replacing the estimated fluid deficit within 3 or 4 hours of initial presentation. In patients with severe dehydration, isotonic intravenous fluids should be used, and lactated Ringer's solution is the preferred commercially available option. For patients without severe dehydration, oral rehydration solution is the standard.

b. Prompt initiation of antimicrobial therapy decreases the duration and volume of diarrhea and decreases the shedding of viable bacteria. Antimicrobial therapy is recommended only for people who are moderately to severely ill. Table 18 shows the antibiotics for treatment of suspected cholera.

Prevention

a. There is one cholera vaccine available for use in the United States. Pre-exposure prophylaxis is recommended for persons 2 to 64 years of age traveling to cholera-affected countries.

b. The vaccine is a live, attenuated vaccine that is taken as a single, oral liquid dose (~3 fl oz.) at least 10 days prior to traveling to a cholera-affected area to protect against disease caused by *V. cholerae* serogroup O1.

c. Most common reported adverse reactions are tiredness, headache, abdominal pain, nausea/vomiting, lack of appetite, and diarrhea.

Table 18 ANTIBIOTICS FOR TREATMENT OF SUSPECTED CHOLERA

Antibiotic	Pediatric Dose	Adult Dose
Azithromycin	20 mg/kg, single dose	1 g, single dose
Ciprofloxacin[a]	15 mg/kg, twice daily × 3 days	500 mg, twice daily × 3 days
Doxycycline[b]	4–6 mg/kg, single dose	300 mg, single dose
Erythromycin	12.5 mg/kg, 4 times/day × 3 days	250 mg, 4 times/day × 3 days
Tetracycline	12.5 mg/kg, 4 times/day × 3 days	500 mg, 4 times/day × 3 days

[a]Ciprofloxacin is not usually recommended in children or pregnant women but may be used if needed.
[b]Doxycycline is not recommended in children younger than age 8 years or in pregnant women.

Duration of Protection and Efficacy

Unknown. Randomized, placebo-controlled human challenge studies (challenged by oral ingestion of *V. cholerae*) demonstrated an efficacy of 90.3% among persons challenged 10 days post-vaccination and 80% among those challenged 3 months post-vaccination.

Contraindications and Precautions for Cholera Vaccine

Contraindications
1. Persons with a history of severe allergic reaction (e.g., anaphylaxis) to any ingredient of this cholera vaccine or to a previous dose of any cholera vaccine

Precautions
1. The safety and effectiveness have not been established in immunocompromised persons or persons receiving immunosuppressive therapies. Vaccine strain may be shed in the stool of recipients for at least 7 days. There is a potential for transmission of the vaccine strain to nonvaccinated close contacts.
2. The safety and effectiveness have not been established in children younger than age 2 years or in adults older than age 65 years.

Frequently Asked Questions

Where do cholera outbreaks occur?
Cholera outbreaks occur in areas where there are natural disasters or in situations in which there is a loss of sanitary human waste disposal and lack of clean water and foods for people to eat. In low-income countries, hunger can lead people to eat contaminated food and/or drink contaminated water, which increases the risk for cholera to infect malnourished populations.

Are there persons who are at higher risk to become infected with cholera than others?
Yes. People who are malnourished or immune compromised and children aged 2 to 4 years are more likely to become infected. Also, people with blood type O are twice as likely to develop cholera, and people with achlorhydria (reduced acid secretion in the stomach) or persons taking medications to reduce stomach acid (e.g., H2 blockers) are more likely to develop cholera because stomach acid kills the cholera organism.

How contagious is cholera?
It takes approximately 100 million *V. cholerae* bacteria to infect a healthy adult. Because this number is so high, significant contamination of food or water is required to transmit the disease. In outbreaks, cholera-causing bacteria become highly contagious indirectly and directly by the fecal–oral route because of widespread fecal contamination of food, water, and items such as bedding and clothing.

TICK-BORNE ENCEPHALITIS VACCINE

Did you know that:

- The Central European countries account for the highest number of cases of tick-borne encephalitis during the highest period of tick activity from April to November.
- Tick-borne encephalitis is more common in adults than in children.
- One in three people may have long-term effects that may last months to years, including cognitive changes and muscle weakness, or permanent paralysis.

Tick-borne encephalitis (TBE) is a human viral infection of the central nervous system (brain and spinal cord) that occurs in many areas of Central Europe and several regions in Asia. It is caused by a tick-borne encephalitis virus (TBEV) of the *Flavivirus* genus that has three subtypes: Far Eastern, Siberian, and European. It is transmitted to humans through the bite of an infected tick (*Ixodes ricinus, Ixodes persulcatus, Ixodes ovatus*) and less commonly by ingestion of unpasteurized milk or milk products from infected livestock, particularly goats. TBE can affect people of all ages who come into contact with ticks during recreational or occupational outdoor activities in woodland habitats of countries where ticks infected with TBE virus are prevalent. Adults account for the majority of cases. TBEV is considered endemic in 27 European countries and highly endemic in Belarus, Czech Republic, Estonia, southern Germany, Latvia, Lithuania, Poland, Russia, Siberia, Slovenia, Switzerland, and northeastern China.

The neurotropic TBEV was first described as the cause of TBE by L. A. Zilber more than 85 years ago. TBE has become a growing public health challenge in Europe and other areas of the world. The number of human cases of TBE in all endemic areas of Europe has increased by almost 400% in the past 30 years, with an expansion in the areas of risk. In Europe and Asia, there are upwards of 15,000 cases reported annually. With the significant increase in tourism and international travel, TBE has become a more global issue.

Approximately two-thirds of human TBE virus infections are asymptomatic. In symptomatic cases, TBE usually has a biphasic course. The first viremic phase lasts approximately 5 days (range: 2–10 days) and is associated with nonspecific symptoms such as fever, fatigue, nausea, headache, and myalgias. This phase is followed by an asymptomatic interval lasting 7 days (range: 1–33 days). This is followed by the development of symptoms of central nervous system involvement (meningitis, meningoencephalitis, myelitis, radiculitis, and paralysis), with meningitis and meningoencephalitis being the most frequent clinical forms of TBE. Disease tends to be more severe in older individuals and immunocompromised persons. Meningitis typically manifests with high fever, headache, nausea, vomiting, photophobia, and some vertigo. Meningoencephalitis may manifest with impaired consciousness, personality changes, behavioral disorders, concentration and cognitive function disturbances, tongue fasciculations, tremor of the extremities, and flaccid paralysis. Rarely, persons may also have delirium, focal or generalized seizures, and psychosis. There is no specific antiviral treatment for TBE. Treatment of hospitalized patients is supportive care.

Transmission

1. Bite of an infected *I. ricinus*, *I. persulcatus*, or *I. ovatus* tick
2. Ingestion of unpasteurized milk or milk products from infected livestock animals, particularly goats

Incubation Period

The incubation period of TBE ranges from 2 to 28 days and is usually 7 to 14 days. For alimentary TBEV acquisition, the incubation period is shorter, usually 3 or 4 days.

Prevention

1. Vaccination against TBE with inactivated whole virus vaccine which may be used in persons 1 year of age or older. Vaccine is given as a 0.5 mL intramuscular injection. The vaccination schedule is as follows:

Age of Person	Primary Vaccination Schedule			
	Dose 1	Dose 2	Dose 3	Booster
Children (1–15 years)	Day 0	14 days to 3 months after dose 1	5–12 months after dose 2	A fourth dose may be given at least 3 years after completion of the primary schedule if ongoing exposure or re-exposure to TBE is expected.
Adults (≥16 years)	Day 0	1–3 months after dose 1	5–12 months after dose 2	

2. Application of insect repellents
3. Wearing protective clothing with long sleeves and long pants tucked into socks treated with an appropriate insecticide

Duration of Protection

After the third primary series dose, duration of protection is at least 3 years. A fourth dose may be given at least 3 years after completion of the primary schedule if ongoing exposure or re-exposure to TBE is expected.

Contraindications and Precautions to Tick-Borne Encephalitis Vaccine

Contraindications
1. Severe allergic reaction (e.g., anaphylaxis) after a previous dose or to a vaccine component

Precautions
1. Moderate or severe acute illness with or without fever

Frequently Asked Questions

Which travelers to Europe and Asia should receive TBE vaccine?
The risk for TBE for the majority of U.S. travelers visiting TBE endemic areas in Europe and Asia is very low. However, some people who travel abroad to TBE endemic areas are at increased risk for infection based on timing of travel during the warmer spring and summer months, travel location, participation in certain recreational outdoor activities (e.g., fishing, hunting, camping, and hiking) in tick habitats in or on the edges of forests, working in outdoor settings where there is the increased potential of coming into contact with infected ticks (e.g., farmers, forestry workers, military personnel, and researchers undertaking field work), and staying for longer periods of time or repeated travel to endemic areas. These individuals should be advised to take precautions to avoid tick bites, and TBE vaccine should be recommended.

Am I at risk for TBE if I plan to travel to Estonia during the summer for several weeks and will visit a farm that has horses, cows, and goats?
Estonia is a country in Europe that is considered highly endemic for TBE. TBE is most commonly transmitted to humans through the bite of an infected tick; however, less commonly it can be transmitted by ingestion of unpasteurized milk or milk products from infected livestock animals, particularly goats. If you plan to visit the farm, do not ingest any

unpasteurized milk or milk products (e.g., yogurt, cheese, and ice cream) because doing so will increase your risk for TBE. Given that you are traveling to a highly endemic country during a time of year when there is high tick activity and you are staying there for a length of time, you should protect yourself and your family by getting TBE vaccine.

REFERENCES

Bogovic P, Strle F. Tick-borne encephalitis: A review of epidemiology, clinical characteristics, and management. *World J Clin Cases*. 2015;3(5):430–441.

Centers for Disease Control and Prevention. Tick-borne encephalitis. n.d. https://www.cdc.gov/tick-borne-encephalitis

European Centre for Disease Prevention and Control. Factsheet about tick-borne encephalitis (TBE). n.d. https://www.ecdc.europa.eu/en/tick-borne-encephalitis/facts/factsheet

INDEX

For the benefit of digital users, indexed terms that span two pages (e.g., 52–53) may, on occasion, appear on only one of those pages.

Tables, figures, and boxes are indicated by an italic *t*, *f*, and *b* following the page number.

ACAM2000, smallpox vaccine against mpox, 250, 252–53
active immunization, 1
adolescents
  immunization schedule, 26*f*
  meningococcal vaccines, 192
  notes on child/adolescent immunization schedule, 29*f*
  pertussis complications, 88–90
  pertussis evaluation, 88
  recommended catch-up immunization schedule, 27*f*
  recommended immunization schedule by medical indication, 28*f*
  serogroup B meningococcal vaccines, 192–93
  sexual activity and HPV vaccination, 199
  signs and symptoms of pertussis in, 87*t*
adults
  complications of influenza, 101–2
  Hib vaccines, 207
  immunization schedules by age group, 37*f*
  immunization schedules by medication condition/indication, 38*f*
  MMR vaccine dose recommendations, 144–45
  notes on recommended immunization by age, 39*f*
  pertussis complications, 88–90
  pertussis evaluation, 88
  recombinant, adjuvanted zoster vaccine to, over 50 years, 168–69
  rotavirus infection, 221
  signs and symptoms of pertussis in, 87*t*
  summary of vaccines routinely recommended for, 47*t*
  Tdap vaccine administration, 96
  yellow fever vaccination, 260
Advisory Committee on Immunization Practices (ACIP), Centers for Disease Control and Prevention (CDC), 3, 59

INDEX

Aedes aegypti
 dengue transmission, 243, 244
 yellow fever transmission, 255, 257
Aedes albopictus, dengue transmission, 243, 244
Affordable Care Act, vaccine coverage, 3
age
 administration of pneumococcal vaccines, 179
 pneumococcal vaccines for adults of 19-64, 176
 pneumococcal vaccines for adults of 65 and older, 176
 recombinant, adjuvanted zoster vaccine, 168
 vaccine dose administration, 2
 vaccine injection site and needle size, 24t
Alda, Alan, polio, 208
American Academy of Family Physicians (AAFP), immunization of pregnant women, 79
American Academy of Pediatrics, 19, 64, 85-86
 AAP Committee on Infectious Diseases, 106-7
American Congress of Obstetricians and Gynecologists (ACOG), 59, 62, 64
 immunization of pregnant women, 79
 quadrivalent inactivated influenza vaccine (IIV4), 105
antibiotics
 health care workers and pertussis, 94
 meningococcal disease, 186, 187t
 treatment of suspected cholera, 280t
 treatment for pertussis, 89t
 vaccine-preventable infections, 15-16
antiviral medications, influenza vaccination, 108
arthritis, MMR vaccine and, 151
aseptic meningitis, 209
asthma, influenza vaccination, 108
autism spectrum disorder (ASD), 4-6, 7-8
 causes of, 8
 health care provider communication tips, 8-9

measles, mumps, rubella (MMR) and, 7
 misconception on vaccines and, 7-9
 MMR vaccine and, 7-8
 MMR vaccine or thimerosal and, 150-51

bacterial meningitis, *Hemophilus influenzae* type b (Hib), 202
Barr, Roseann, herpes zoster (shingles), 164
barriers, adolescent and adult immunization, 5t
Black Death (bubonic plague), 99
blood donation, hepatitis A virus, 123
body mass, vaccine injection site and needle size, 24t
bone marrow transplant
 influenza vaccine, 113
 Tdap vaccine, 85
booster dose
 cocoon effect for Tdap booster, 97
 DTaP vaccine for children, 98
 Japanese encephalitis, 269
 Meningococcal for 3- or 5-year, 194
 mpox, 252
 Tdap vaccine, 96
 tetanus, 96
breastfed infant, MMR vaccine and, 140
breastfeeding mothers
 HbsAg-positive, 132
 MMR vaccine and, 140
 Tdap vaccine, 97
Bronson, Charles, pneumococcal pneumonia, 171
Brown, James, pneumococcal pneumonia, 171

Candy Land (game), polio, 209
Carver, George Washington, 85
catarrhal stage, pertussis, 86
CDC SHARE program, 6-233
 addressing, 232-33
 explaining, 233
 highlighting, 232
 reminding, 233
 sharing, 232

INDEX

Centers for Disease Control and Prevention (CDC), xi, 64
ACAM2000 not recommended for, 253
Advisory Committee on Immunization Practices (ACIP), 3, 59
ASD and vaccine study, 7–8
definition of close contacts, 89–90
egg-allergic patients and influenza, 106–7
evidence of immunity to measles, mumps, and rubella, 139
HPV infections in United States, 194–95
immunization of pregnant women, 79
infant, child and adolescent immunization schedules, 26f
meningococcal disease and pregnancy, 67–68
notes on child/adolescent immunization schedule, 29f
pneumococcal vaccine-naïve persons, 175–76
post-exposure protection against hepatitis A, 124–25
recommendation for mumps patients, 144
recommendations for MMR to infants for international travel, 140
recommended catch-up immunization schedule, 27f
recommended child and adolescent immunization schedule by medical indication, 28f
safety of vaccines, 13
studies of MMR vaccine and ASD, 150–51
Tdap vaccine, 93
tetanus toxoid-containing vaccines for refugees/immigrants, 97–98
varicella immunity in health care personnel, 162
varicella vaccine recommendations, 160
cervical cancer, HPV vaccine and, 200
Charlie and the Chocolate Factory (Dahl), 134
chemoprophylaxis
 Hemophilus influenzae type b (Hib), 203–4
 pertussis treatment for close contacts, 88–90
chemotherapy
 MMR vaccine to sibling of child receiving, 140
 recombinant, adjuvanted zoster vaccine (Shingrix) and, 170
chickenpox
 disease before first birthday and varicella vaccine, 159
 mild case and immunity, 160
 natural and vaccine-acquired immunity, 11
 recombinant, adjuvanted zoster vaccine for adults over 50, 168–69
 varicella vaccine and, 160
 varicella vaccine and exposure, 159
 See also varicella zoster
children
 DTaP instead of Tdap, 95
 DTaP vaccine booster, 98
 immunization schedule, 26f
 influenza vaccine and, 116
 notes on child/adolescent immunization schedule, 29f
 pertussis complications, 88–90
 pneumococcal vaccine PPSV23, 177–78
 pneumococcal vaccines, 177
 recommended catch-up immunization schedule, 27f
 recommended immunization schedule by medical indication, 28f
 summary of vaccines routinely recommended for, 47t
chimpanzee coryza agent (CCA), 235
 See also respiratory syncytial virus (RSV)
cholera
 antibiotics for treating suspected, 280t
 antimicrobial therapy, 279
 areas of world for outbreaks, 277f
 contagion of, 282
 contraindications of vaccine, 280
 diarrhea of, 276
 duration of protection, 280
 efficacy of vaccine, 280

291

INDEX

cholera (cont.)
  frequently asked questions, 281–82
  incubation period, 278
  infection and death, 276
  manifestation of, 278
  outbreaks, 281
  precautions of vaccine, 281
  pregnancy and vaccine, 60t, 65
  prevention, 279
  rehydration therapy, 276, 279
  risk of persons for, 281
  transmission, 278
  treatment, 279
  Vibrio cholerae, 276–78, 279, 280, 282
chronic disease, hepatitis A virus, 121
Clarke, Arthur C., polio, 208
close contact(s)
  definition by CDC, 89–90
  meningococcal disease transmission, 185–86
Clostridium tetani, 79, 80
cochlear implant
  pneumococcal vaccines and, 182
  risk for pneumococcal disease, 173
cocoon effect, Tdap booster, 97
cocoon strategy, protecting infants, 85–86
combination vaccines, dose and route of administration, 21t
Comirnaty, COVID-19, 230
commonly used vaccines, contradictions and precautions, 223, 223t
congenital rubella syndrome (CRS), risk of developing, 65, 71
convalescent stage, pertussis, 87
Corynebacterium diphtheria, 74, 75
COVID-19, 20t, 228–35
  adverse effects, 231–32
  age group and dosing, 47t
  contraindications of vaccines, 232–33
  dose and route for administration, 21t
  frequently asked questions, 233–35
  incubation period, 229
  infertility and vaccination, 234
  ingredients in vaccine, 234
  long COVID, 230

  mRNA vaccines, 63, 230
  notes on adult immunization schedule, 39f
  notes on child/adolescent immunization schedule, 29f
  pandemic, 228
  post-COVID-19 syndrome, 230
  post-exposure vaccination, 234
  precautions of vaccines, 233
  pregnancy and, 60t, 62–63
  prevention, 230
  risk factors for getting very sick, 63
  SARS-CoV-2 (severe acute respiratory syndrome coronavirus 2), 58, 229
  transmission, 229
  vaccination recommendations, 63
  vaccinations and pregnancy, 234
  Vaccine Adverse Event Reporting System (VAERS), 234–35
  vaccine inequity, 232
  viral mutation, 233

Dahl, Roald, measles death, 134
day care setting, hepatitis B virus, 130
day care workers, hepatitis A vaccine, 122
Democratic Republic of the Congo (DRC), mpox infected infant, 247
dengue, 20t, 243–47
  contraindications for vaccine, 245–46
  Dengvaxia (vaccine), 245
  dose and route for administration, 21t
  duration of immunity, 245
  epidemics, 243
  frequently asked questions, 246–47
  incubation period, 244
  infection with, 243–44
  notes on child/adolescent immunization schedule, 29f
  pregnancy and vaccine, 60t, 65–66
  precautions for vaccine, 246
  prevention, 245, 247
  reinfection, 246
  transmission, 244
  traveling and vaccination, 246
  treatment, 244

INDEX

vaccine efficacy, 245
viral serotypes (DENV-1, DENV-2, DENV-3, and DENV-4), 243, 246
word, 243
Dengvaxia, dengue vaccine, 245
Descartes, Rene, pneumococcal pneumonia, 171
diphtheria, ix, 2, 73–78
   cases and deaths in 1921 (United States), 73
   consequences of being untreated for, 78
   contagious period, 78
   contraindications to vaccines containing, 76
   Corynebacterium diphtheria, 74, 75
   death of Dr. Jacobi's son, 73
   description of, 74
   duration of immunity, 76
   frequently asked questions, 77–78
   historic descriptions, 73
   immunity, 78
   incubation period, 75
   life-threatening complications, 74
   post-exposure, 75
   precautions to vaccines containing, 77
   pre-exposure, 76
   prevalence and risk, 77
   prevention, 75–76
   risk of acquiring, 77
   transmission, 75
diphtheria, tetanus, pertussis (combination vaccines)
   age group and dosing (DTaP), 47*t*
   booster for children (DTaP), 98
   contraindications and precautions, 223*t*
   dose and route for administration, 21*t*
   doses of pediatric, 94
   encephalopathy (DTaP), 92
   notes on child/adolescent immunization schedule, 29*f*
   persistent crying (DTaP), 95–96
   pertussis containing vaccines (DTaP), 90, 91
   precautions (DTaP), 92–93
   tetanus immunization, 82
   wound management and immunization history, 81, 81*t*
   See also diphtheria; pertussis; tetanus
Doolittle, James H., herpes zoster (shingles), 164
DTaP-IPB-Hib (Pentacel), dose and route of administration, 21*t*
DTaP-IPV (Kinrix; Quadracel), dose and route of administration, 21*t*
DTaP-IPV-HepB (Pediarix), dose and route of administration, 21*t*
DTaP-IPV-Hib-HepB (Vaxelis), dose and route of administration, 21*t*

Ebola, 20*t*
Effendi, Shoghi, 99
egg allergy
   influenza patients with, 106–7
   influenza vaccine, 111
   MMR vaccine and, 140
elderly individuals
   high-dose influenza vaccine and, 113, 116
   influenza vaccine and, 112
   yellow fever vaccine, 260
elective splenectomy, Hib vaccines, 207
Engerix-B, hepatitis B vaccine, 134
environmental stability
   hepatitis A virus, 121
   hepatitis B virus, 130–31
epididymo-orchitis, mumps complication, 141
ethylmercury, thimerosal and, 12–13
Expanded Access Investigational New Drug, ACAM2000 for use against mpox, 250

Farrow, Mia, polio, 208
father of American pediatrics, Abraham Jacobi, 73
fetal mortality, mumps, 142
flavivirus, Japanese encephalitis virus, 266
Flavivirus, dengue, 243
Flavivirus, tick-borne encephalitis virus (TBEV), 282–83

INDEX

flu. *See* influenza
FluMist Quadrivalent, influenza vaccines, 105–6
flu vaccine
  benefits of, 109
  pregnancy and, 70
  value of high-dose, 111
Franklin, Benjamin. vaccination advice, 3–4
Franklin, Francis Folger. smallpox death, 3–4
frequently asked questions
  cholera, 281–82
  dengue, 246–47
  diphtheria, 77–78
  hepatitis A virus, 121–25
  hepatitis B virus, 130–34
  herpes zoster (shingles), 168–70
  human papillomavirus (HPV) vaccines, 198–201
  influenza, 109–16
  Japanese encephalitis (JE), 269–70
  measles, 138–40
  meningococcal disease and vaccines, 191–94
  MMR (measles, mumps, rubella) vaccine, 138–40
  mpox, 252–54
  mumps and MMR vaccine, 144–45
  pertussis, 93–98
  pneumococcal vaccines, 177–82
  poliovirus vaccination, 213–16
  pregnancy and vaccines, 70–71
  rabies, 275
  respiratory syncytial virus (RSV), 240–42
  rubella and MMR vaccine, 149–51
  tetanus, 83–85
  typhoid fever, 264–65
  varicella (chickenpox) vaccine, 159–64
  yellow fever vaccine, 259–60

German measles, 145–46
  See also rubella
Guillain-Barré syndrome (GBS)
  influenza vaccination and, 108, 110

quadrivalent inactivated influenza vaccine (IIV4), 105
tetanus toxoid-containing vaccine, 92

H1N1 influenza A, pandemic (2009), 58, 99, 102
Haemophilus influenzae type b (Hib) vaccine. *See* Hemophilus influenzae type B (Hib) vaccine
Harrison, Benjamin, 99
health care provider(s)
  antibiotic prophylaxis, 94
  CDC recommending recombinant, adjuvanted zoster vaccine, 168
  hepatitis A vaccine, 122
  influenza vaccine, 114
  live, attenuated influenza vaccine (LAIV), 114
  tetanus-containing vaccines, 84
  tetanus-diphtheria-acellular pertussis (Tdap) vaccine, 93
  vaccine recommendations, 6–233
  varicella vaccine and, 162
  zoster vaccine, 162
Healthy People 2030, x, 101
Hemophilus influenzae type B (Hib) vaccine, 20t
  adults, 207
  age group and dosing, 47t
  children and, 206–7
  contraindications, 205, 223t
  dose and route for administration, 21t
  efficacy, 205
  elective splenectomy, 207
  frequently asked questions, 205–7
  GSK monovalent product (Hiberix), 206
  impact of vaccination, 15–16
  infants and, 206–7
  notes on adult immunization schedule, 39f
  notes on child/adolescent immunization schedule, 29f
  post-exposure, 204
  precautions, 205, 223t
  pre-exposure, 205

INDEX

Hemophilus influenzae type B disease, 201–7
  chemoprophylaxis, 203–4
  Hib vaccine, 204, 205
  H. influenzae type b (Hib) as pleomorphic gram-negative coccobacillus, 202
  incubation period, 203
  infection before vaccine availability, 201
  Pfeiffer isolating bacterium, 201–2
  post-exposure, 203–4
  pre-exposure, 205
  prevention, 203–5
  rifampin chemoprophylaxis for contacts of index cases, 203–4
  risk factors for, 202–3
  transmission, 203
HepA-HepB (Twinrix), dose and route of administration, 21t
hepatitis A, 7–8, 20t
  dose and route for administration, 21t
  epidemic of, 117
  immunogenicity, 120
  incubation period, 119
  post-exposure, 119–20
  pre-exposure, 120
  pregnancy and, 60t, 66
  prevention, 119–20
  recommendations for vaccination, 119–20
  transmission, 119
  vaccination introduction, 117–19
  vaccine, 120
hepatitis A vaccine, 7–8
  administering an extra dose, 124
  adults receiving pediatric dose, 122–23
  age group and dosing, 47t
  blood donation and, 123
  breastfeeding women, 122
  CDC guidelines for post-exposure protection, 124–25
  childcare centers, 122
  contraindications, 120
  duration of protection, 120
  frequently asked questions, 121–25
  notes on adult immunization schedule, 39f
  notes on child/adolescent immunization schedule, 29f
  precautions, 121
  prevaccination testing before administration, 121
  protection from, 123
  travel abroad, 123–24
hepatitis A virus (HAV)
  blood donation and, 123
  chronic disease, 121
  health care workers (HCWs), 122
  post-exposure prophylaxis (PEP) after exposure, 124
  post-vaccination testing, 122
  stability in environment, 121
hepatitis B surface antigen (HBsAg), 66–67
  breastfeeding by HbsAg-positive mother, 132
  mother's test and managing infant, 131–32
  person receiving HBV vaccine with negative HbsAg, 133–34
hepatitis B vaccine, 7–8, 20t
  age group and dosing, 47t
  contraindications, 130
  contraindications and precautions, 223t
  dose and route for administration, 21t
  duration of protection, 129
  efficacy, 129
  infants receiving adult dose, 132–33
  notes on adult immunization schedule, 39f
  notes on child/adolescent immunization schedule, 29f
  post-vaccination serologic testing, 133
  precautions, 130
  pregnancy and, 60t, 66–67
  using different brands of, 134
hepatitis B virus (HBV), 125–34
  age at time of infection as risk of chronic infection, 127
  CDC estimate of annual cases in United States, 125–26

INDEX

hepatitis B virus (HBV) (*cont.*)
  death, 125
  frequently asked questions, 130–34
  incubation period, 127–28
  infection, 125
  post-exposure, 128–29
  pre-exposure, 129
  prevention, 128–29
  reinfection occurrence, 130
  risk factors for, 126–27
  screening blood test for pregnant women, 131
  signs and symptoms, 125–26
  stability in environment, 130–31
  transmission, 127
  worldwide infection, 125
herd immunity, 17
herpes, Greek word, 164
herpes zoster (shingles), 164–70
  age group and dosing of vaccine, 47*t*
  CDC recommending recombinant, adjuvanted zoster vaccine, 168
  clinical features, 165
  complications, 165–66
  contraindications of vaccine, 168
  duration of protection, 167
  effectiveness of Shingrix, 167
  frequently asked questions, 168–70
  neurocutaneous disease, 164–65
  precautions of vaccine, 168
  prevention, 167
  Shingrix, 20*t*
  term, 164
  transmission, 166
Hib-HepB (Comvax), dose and route of administration, 21*t*
Hib-MenCY (MenHibrix), dose and route of administration, 21*t*
Hippocrates, description of mumps, 141
hospital employees, varicella vaccine and, 161–62
human papillomavirus (HPV), 7–8, 20*t*, 194–201
  contraindications of vaccine, 198, 223*t*
  disease manifestations, 195
  dose and route for administration, 21*t*
  duration of immunity, 198
  frequently asked questions, 198–201
  immunogenicity, 197–98
  incidence, 194
  incubation period, 196
  infection, 194–95
  post-exposure, 196–97
  precautions of vaccine, 198, 223*t*
  pre-exposure, 197
  prevention, 196–97
  serotypes, 195
  transmission, 195–96
human papillomavirus (HPV) vaccine(s), 197
  age group and dosing, 47*t*
  contraindications and precautions, 198
  HPV2 or HPV4, 198–200
  HPV9, 197, 198–200
  immunogenicity, 197–98
  notes on adult immunization schedule, 39*f*
  notes on child/adolescent immunization schedule, 29*f*
  pregnancy and, 199
  sexual activity in teenagers, 199
  subcutaneous and intramuscular route, 201
hygiene and sanitation, vaccine-preventable infections, 15–16

immigrants, vaccine schedule, 97–98
immune globulin (IG), post-exposure protection against hepatitis A, 124–25
immune system, misconception about infants', 9–10
immunity, measles for those born before 1957, 138
immunization
  active, 1
  barriers to adolescent and adult, 5*t*
  passive, 1
  public health initiative, ix
Immunization Action Coalition, 19

INDEX

immunization schedules
  adult, 37f
  break in vaccine, 2
  infant, child and adolescent, 26f
  recommended child and adolescent, by medical indication, 28f
immunocompromised persons
  influenza, 108
  varicella vaccine in, 161
  yellow fever vaccine, 259
immunodeficiency
  live, attenuated vaccines and, 3
  varicella vaccine in children, 161
immunologic response, vaccine, 2
immunosuppressive chemotherapy, zoster vaccine and, 170
Imovax, human diploid cell vaccine, 273
inactivated polio virus (IPV) vaccine, 20t
  age group and dosing, 47t
  contraindications and precautions, 223t
  pre-exposure prophylaxis, 211–12, 214–16
  pregnant women, 68
inactivated vaccines, common, 20t
infants
  cocoon strategy for protecting, 85–86
  DTaP vaccine for, 94
  health care provider communication tips, 10
  hepatitis B vaccine, 132–33
  immunization schedule, 26f
  misconception about immune system of, 9–10
  mother's HBsAg test status, 131–32
  pertussis (whooping cough) in, 60–61
  pneumococcal vaccines, 177
  respiratory syncytial virus (RSV), 71
  rotavirus infection and vaccination, 221
  rotavirus vaccination, 221–22
  rotavirus vaccine schedule, 221
  summary of vaccines routinely recommended for, 47t
  Tdap and pediatric DTaP, 94–95
  transmission of varicella virus, 160–61

unprotected worldwide, ix–x
varicella vaccine, 159
varicella zoster immune globulin (VariZIG), 163–64
infertility, COVID-19 vaccines and, 234
influenza, 98–117
  age group and dosing, 47t
  annual epidemics, 99–100
  clinical presentation, 100
  complications in adult population, 101–2
  duration of protection, 107
  efficacy, 107
  egg-allergic patients, 106–7
  frequently asked questions, 109–16
  H1N1 pandemic (2009), 99
  incubation period, 102
  persons at risk for complications, 100–1
  post-exposure, 103–4
  pre-exposure, 104–6
  pregnancy and, 60t, 61–62
  pregnant women, 102
  prevention, 103–6
  Spanish pandemic (1918), 99
  transmission, 102
  vaccines, 104–6
  word, 98–99
influenza pandemic (1917-1918), 58
influenza vaccine(s), 7–8
  contraindications, 107–8
  contraindications and precautions (IIV), 223t
  contraindications and precautions (LAIV), 223t
  contraindications and precautions (RIV) (Flublok), 223t
  dose and route for administration (IIV), 21t
  dose and route for administration (LAIV), 21t
  egg-based, 114
  FluMist Quadrivalent, 105–6
  Guillain-Barré syndrome (GBS) and, 110
  high-dose, and persons over 65 years, 113

influenza vaccine(s) (*cont.*)
  immunity and strains, 110
  immunity from seasonal, 109–10
  inactivated, quadrivalent (IIV4), 105
  inactivated, quadrivalent (IIV4), high dose, 104, 105
  inactivated, quadrivalent cell culture-based (ccIIV4), 104, 105
  inactivated, quadrivalent egg-based (IIV4e), 104
  inactivated, quadrivalent egg-based adjuvanted with MF59 (aIIV4), 104
  injectable inactivated (IIV), 106–7
  international travel and, 116
  live, attenuated, quadrivalent (LAIV4), 104, 106–7
  misconception on "getting the flu" from, 112–13
  notes on adult immunization schedule, 39*f*
  notes on child/adolescent immunization schedule, 29*f*
  patient believing they had a reaction to, 115–16
  precautions, 108
  protection from seasonal, 109
  protective immunity, 112–13
  providers offering, 110
  recombinant (RIV4), 104
  recombinant influenza vaccine (RIV), 105–6
  traveling abroad, 116
  vaccines containing thimerosal (IIV), 14*t*
injectable influenza, 20*t*
injectable typhoid fever, 20*t*
Institute of Medicine (IOM), 7–8
  thimerosal-containing vaccines and ASD, 150–51
international travel
  CDC recommendations for MMR to infants, 140
  infants and varicella vaccine, 159
  influenza vaccine and, 116
  vaccination and, 17
intramuscular (IM) injection
  HPV vaccine and, 201
  injection site and needle size, 24*t*

intranasal influenza, 2, 20*t*
invasive pneumococcal disease (IPD), 171–72
  See also pneumococcal disease
IPV. *See* inactivated polio virus (IPV) vaccine
iron lung, 208
Ixodes ovatus, tick-borne encephalitis (TBE), 282–83, 284
Ixodes persulcatus, TBE, 282–83, 284
Ixodes ricinus, TBE, 282–83, 284

J&J/Janssen COVID-19 vaccine, 230, 232
Jacobi, Abraham, father of American Pediatrics, 73
Japanese encephalitis (JE), 20*t*, 265–70
  booster dose of vaccine, 269
  contraindications of vaccine, 269
  duration of protection, 269
  earliest symptoms of, 266
  frequently asked questions, 269–70
  global areas where serologic groups of, are endemic and epidemic, 267*f*
  incubation, 266
  mosquito larvae infected with JE virus, 265
  precautions of vaccine, 269
  pre-exposure prophylaxis, 268
  pregnancy and, 68
  prevention, 268–69
  seizures, 265
  transmission, 268
  treatment, 268
  vaccine-preventable encephalitis, 265
  virus as flavivirus, 266
JYNNEOS, smallpox vaccine against mpox, 250, 251–53

Kahlo, Frida, polio, 208
Karloff, Boris, pneumococcal pneumonia, 171

Lancet, The (journal), 7
Letterman, David, herpes zoster (shingles), 164
Lincoln, Abraham, death of sons by infectious diseases, 73

INDEX

Lindbergh, Charles, herpes zoster (shingles), 164
live, attenuated influenza vaccine (LAIV)
  breastfeeding and, 115
  health care personnel, 114
  immunosuppressed patients, 115
  respiratory infection, 114
  young patient and half the dose, 115
live, attenuated vaccines
  common, 20t
  contraindications, 3
  MMR (measles, mumps, rubella), 65
  oral cholera vaccine, 69–70
  persons who should not receive LAIV (influenza vaccine), 112
  tetravalent dengue vaccine, 70
live, attenuated zoster vaccine, (Zostavax), 167, 169
  discontinuation of, 169
Lives of a Cell, The (Thomas), 270

Madison, Dolly, 85
Madison, James, 85
Mallon, Mary, "Typhoid Mary", 260–61
measles, ix, 134–40
  complications, 135–36
  duration of protection, 138
  frequently asked questions, 138–40
  immunity for people born before 1957, 138
  immunogenicity, 137
  incubation period, 136
  infection during pregnancy, 136
  natural and vaccine-acquired immunity, 11
  post-exposure, 136–37
  pre-exposure, 137
  pregnancy and, 64
  prevention, 136–37
  Staphylococcus aureus, 135–36
  Streptococcus pneumoniae, 135–36
  subacute sclerosing panencephalitis (SSPE), 135–36
  transmission, 135, 136
  vaccination rates, 136
  virus, 135
  worldwide deaths, 135

See also MMR (measles, mumps, rubella) vaccine
Medical Library Association, 19
Meir, Golda, herpes zoster (shingles), 164
meningitis, complications of, 184
meningitis belt, 182–83
Meningitis Vaccine Project, 182–83
meningococcal B (MenB), 20t
  age group and dosing, 47t
meningococcal disease, 182–94
  antibiotic chemoprophylaxis, 186
  clinical presentations, 183–84
  common serogroups causing, 185
  complications and sequelae, 184–85
  conjugate meningococcal type A vaccine, 182–83
  frequently asked questions, 191–94
  incubation period, 186
  "meningitis belt", 182–83
  meningococcal chemoprophylaxis, 186, 187t
  Neisseria meningitidis causing, 183–85
  onset, 184
  post-exposure, 186
  pre-exposure, 186–90
  pregnancy and, 60t, 67–68
  prevention, 186–90
  recommendations for vaccination, 191–92
  risk factors for, 184–85
  schedule for routine vaccine dosing of adolescents, 187t
  sepsis and, 183
  transmission, 185–86
meningococcal meningitis, epidemics of, 182–83
meningococcal vaccines, 7–8
  age group and dosing (MenACWY), 47t
  age group and dosing (PENBRAYA), 47t
  available conjugate vaccines, 189t
  contraindications of, 191
  dose and route of administration (MCV4), 21t
  dose and route of administration (MCV5), 21t
  dose and route of administration (serogroup B), 21t

INDEX

meningococcal vaccines (cont.)
  doses beyond 3- or 5-year booster, 194
  duration of immunity, 191
  efficacy, 190
  MCV4, 20t, 21t, 191–92
  MCV5, 191
  MenABCWY, 190, 192
  MenACWY, 190
  MenB, 190, 191, 192, 193–94
  MenB-4C (Bexsero), 189–90, 193
  MenB-FHbp (Trumenba), 189–90, 193
  MenHibrix, 189t, 191
  meningococcal serogroup B vaccine (MenB), 189–90
  notes on adult immunization schedule, 39f
  notes on child/adolescent immunization schedule (serogroup A,C,W,Y), 29f
  notes on child/adolescent immunization schedule (serogroup B), 29f
  pentavalent meningococcal conjugate vaccine (MenABCWY), 190
  precautions of, 191
  quadrivalent meningococcal conjugate vaccine (MenACWY), 186–88, 189t
  schedule for routine dosing of adolescents with, 187t
meningococcemia, complications of, 184
mercury, thimerosal, 12–13
Mesopotamian Laws of Eshnunna, rabies, 270
Miranda, Lin-Manuel, herpes zoster (shingles), 164
misconceptions. *See* patient concerns about vaccines
Mitchell, Joni, polio, 208
MMR (measles, mumps, rubella) vaccine, 20t, 21t
  administration after delivery, 150
  administration after reconstituting with diluent, 151
  age group and dosing, 47t
  arthritis and, 151

  autism spectrum disorder (ASD) and, 7, 150–51
  breastfeeding mother or breastfed infant, 140
  contraindications of, 138, 143–44, 223t
  doses for adults, 144–45
  duration of protection, 138
  egg allergy and, 140
  frequently asked questions, 138–40
  intramuscularly (IM) vs. subcutaneously (SC), 139
  mumps post-exposure, 142–43
  mumps pre-exposure, 143
  natural and vaccine-acquired immunity, 11
  notes on adult immunization schedule, 39f
  notes on child/adolescent immunization schedule, 29f
  post-exposure to measles, 137
  precautions of, 138, 223t
  pre-exposure to measles, 137
  pregnancy and, 60t, 65, 149–50
MMRV (measles, mumps, rubella, and varicella) vaccine
  adult vaccination, 139
  dose and route of administration (Proquad), 21t
  MMR vaccine *vs.*, 139
Moderna vaccine, COVID-19, 230, 231
Mohammed Reza Pahlavi (Shah of Iran), 85
Mozart, Wolfgang Amadeus, typhoid fever, 261
mpox, 20t, 247–54
  adverse events, 251
  booster doses, 252
  cases, 248
  CDC recommendations for ACAM2000, 253
  children and vaccination, 253
  contagion of, 252
  DNA virus in *Orthopoxvirus* genus, 248
  dose and route of administration, 21t

INDEX

duration of immunity, 251
epidemic, 248
first documented human case, 247
frequently asked questions, 252–54
incubation period, 249
name monkeypox, 247
pets and, 248, 252
post-exposure vaccination, 249–50
pre-exposure vaccination, 249
prevention, 249–50
reinfection, 254
safety of vaccines, 252–53
smallpox vaccine for, 254
transmission, 248–49
mpox vaccine
  age group and dosing, 47t
  contraindications of vaccines, 251
  licensed smallpox vaccines (ACAM2000 and JYNNEOS), 250, 252–53
  notes on adult immunization schedule, 39f
  notes on child/adolescent immunization schedule, 29f
  precautions of, 251–52
  pregnancy and, 60t, 65
  vaccination candidates, 253
mRNA vaccines, COVID-19, 230
multiple sclerosis
  influenza vaccine, 111
  pneumococcal vaccines and, 182
multisystem inflammatory syndrome in adults (MIS-A), 233
multisystem inflammatory syndrome in children (MIS-C), 233
mumps, 141–45
  complications, 141–42
  contagion period, 144
  contraindications of MMR vaccine, 143–44
  duration of protection, 143
  frequently asked questions, 144–45
  Hippocrates, 141
  immunogenicity, 143
  incubation period, 142
  MMR vaccine, 142
  orchitis and, 141
  post-exposure, 142–43
  precautions of MMR vaccine, 144
  pre-exposure, 143
  pregnancy and, 64–65
  prevention, 142–43
  second occurrences, 144
  systemic disease, 141
  transmission, 142
  See also MMR (measles, mumps, rubella) vaccine

National Network for Immunization Information, 19
natural immunity, misconception about vaccine-acquired immunity and, 11–12
Neisseria meningitidis, 183–84
  causing meningococcal disease, 183–85
  dosing for persons exposed to, 188
neonatal tetanus, 79, 80
Nicklaus, Jack, polio, 208
nirsevimab (Beyfortus), passive immunization for RSV, 238, 242
nutrition, vaccine-preventable infections, 15–16

obstructive sleep apnea (OSA), pneumococcal vaccines, 178–79
oophoritis, mumps complication, 141
oral cholera, 20t
oral live, attenuated polio vaccine (OPV), 212, 213–14, 215, 216
oral typhoid fever, 20t
orchitis, mumps infection, 141
Orthopoxvirus genus, mpox virus, 248
Osler, Sir William, 99

palivizumab (Synagis), passive immunization for RSV, 238–39
Pap tests, HPV vaccine and, 200
paroxysmal stage, pertussis, 87
passive immunization, 1
Pasteur, Louis, *Streptococcus pneumoniae*, 171

301

INDEX

patient barriers, immunization, 5t
patient concerns about vaccines, 3–19
  barriers to adolescent and adult immunization, 5t
  misconception about vaccines causing disease and infection, 18–19
  misconception on autism and vaccines, 7–9
  misconception on infant's immune system, 9–10
  misconception on natural and vaccine-acquired immunity, 11–12
  misconception on risk of, 16–18
  misconception on toxins in vaccines, 12–15
  misconception on vaccine-preventable infections, 15–16
  vaccines containing thimerosal, 14t
pediatric hepatitis A vaccine, adults receiving, 122–23
Peron, Juan, 99
persistent cough, pertussis evaluation, 88
persistent crying
  DTaP vaccine, 95–96
  DTP, DTaP and Tdap vaccines, 95
pertussis (whooping cough), ix, 85–98
  antibiotic prophylaxis, 94
  antibiotic treatment, 89t
  Bordetella pertussis, 85–86
  chemoprophylaxis of close contacts, 88–90, 89t
  clinical signs and symptoms in adolescents and adults, 87t
  close contacts, 89–90
  complications in children, adolescents, and adults, 88–90
  contraindications of vaccine, 92
  duration of immunity, 92
  frequently asked questions, 93–98
  incidence, 85–86
  post-exposure, 90
  precautions of vaccine, 92–93
  pre-exposure, 91
  prevention, 90–91
  reinfection, 93
  severity in infants, 60–61
  stages and severity, 86–87
  transmission, 90
  vaccines containing, 91
  whooping cough, 85–86
pets
  mpox transmission, 248, 252
  rabies, 270
Pfeiffer, Richard, *Hemophilus influenzae* type b (Hib) isolation, 201–2
Pfizer-BioNTech vaccine, COVID-19, 230, 231
physician barriers, immunization, 5t
pneumococcal disease, 171–82
  cases in United States, 171
  conjugate pneumococcal vaccines (PCV7 and PCV13), 171–72
  incubation period, 173
  infection risk, 173
  invasive (IPD), 171–72
  pregnancy and, 60t, 67
  prevention, 173–76
  Streptococcus pneumoniae, 171
  transmission, 172
  vaccine development by Wright, 171
  vaccine efficacy, 176
pneumococcal polysaccharide (PPSV23). *See* pneumococcal vaccines
pneumococcal vaccines
  administration of, 181–82
  age group and dosing (PCV15 and PCV20), 47t
  age group and dosing (PPSV23), 47t
  adults aged 65 and older and vaccination, 180–81
  CDC recommendation, 175–76
  cochlear implant placement, 182
  contraindications and precautions (PCV13), 223t
  contraindications of, 177
  dose and route of administration (PCV), 21t
  dose and route of administration (PPSV23), 21t
  efficacy, 176
  elective splenectomy, 182

INDEX

frequently asked questions, 177–82
multiple sclerosis and, 182
notes on adult immunization schedule, 39f
notes on child/adolescent immunization schedule, 29f
observational studies of (PCV15 and PCV20), 67
observational studies of (PPSV23), 67
PCV13 (13-valent protein conjugate vaccine), 20t, 174–75, 176
PCV15 (15-valent protein conjugate vaccine), 173, 174–75, 176
PCV20 (20-valent protein conjugate vaccine), 173, 174–75, 176
PPSV23 (23-valent polysaccharide vaccine), 20t, 173, 174, 175, 176
precautions of, 177
serotypes of, 179–80
underlying medical conditions and vaccination with, 180–81
polio
near eradication of, ix, 3–4
pregnancy and, 60t, 68
poliomyelitis, 208
adults with paralytic, during childhood, 209
bulbar forms of, 208
epidemic, 208
permanent disability cause, 208
polio vaccine
frequently asked questions, 213–16
inactivated (IPV), 211–12, 214–16
notes on adult immunization schedule, 39f
notes on child/adolescent immunization schedule, 29f
oral live, attenuated (OPV), 212, 213–14, 215, 216
poliovirus(es)
communicability of, 210
group C RNA enteroviruses, 209
types of wild, 208, 209–10
poliovirus infections, 208–16
contraindications of vaccine, 212
duration of immunity, 212

frequently asked questions, 213–16
inactivated polio vaccine (IPV), 211–12, 214–16
incubation period, 210
precautions of vaccine, 213
pre-exposure prophylaxis, 211–12
prevention, 211–12
transmission, 210
vaccine-derived poliovirus (VDPV), 213–14
vaccine efficacy, 212
pork from endemic area, Japanese encephalitis and, 269–70
post-exposure prophylaxis (PEP), hepatitis A virus and, 124
post-polio syndrome, 209
post-vaccination serologic testing, adults with hepatitis B vaccine, 133
post-vaccination testing, hepatitis A virus, 122
pregnancy
COVID-19 vaccines and, 234
flu shot and, 70
HPV vaccine and, 199
live, attenuated vaccines and, 3
measles infection during, 136
MMR vaccine, 149
mumps complication, 142
routine vaccine administration, 59, 60t
Tdap administration, 97
vaccines and, 58–71
yellow fever and, 71
pregnant women
cholera vaccine, 60t, 69–70
COVID-19, 60t, 62–63
dengue vaccine, 60t, 70
frequently asked questions on vaccines, 70–71
hepatitis A, 60t, 66
hepatitis B, 60t, 66–67
hepatitis B vaccine and, 131
influenza, 60t, 61–62, 102, 108
influenza vaccine, 111
Japanese encephalitis, 68
measles, mumps, and rubella (MMR), 60t, 64–65, 149

INDEX

pregnant women (*cont.*)
  meningococcal disease, 60t, 67–68
  mpox vaccine, 60t, 70
  mumps, 64–65
  mumps complications, 142
  pneumococcal disease, 60t, 67
  pneumococcal vaccine PPSV23, 178
  polio, 60t, 68
  rabies, 69
  respiratory syncytial virus (RSV), 60t, 64, 71
  rubella, 65
  rubella test, 149–50
  rubeola (measles), 64
  screening blood test for hepatitis B virus, 131
  screening for HBV, 131
  Tdap (tetanus, diphtheria, acellular pertussis), 59–61, 60t, 96–97
  typhoid fever, 68
  varicella, 60t, 61–62
  yellow fever, 68–69, 71
  yellow fever vaccination, 259–60
prenatal visit, Tdap vaccine and RhoGam immunoglobulin, 85
prevaccination testing, hepatitis A vaccine, 121
prophylactic regimens, treatment for pertussis, 89t
public health, pertussis, 85–86
puncture wounds, tetanus and, 83–84

quadrivalent vaccines. *See* influenza vaccines

RabAvert, rabies vaccine, 273
rabies, 20t
  active prophylaxis, 273
  acute neurologic stage, 270–71
  central nervous system manifestations, 270–71
  contraindications of vaccine, 274
  dogs as main source, 275
  duration of protection, 274
  end of neurologic stage, 270–71
  frequently asked questions, 275
  incubation period, 271
  Mesopotamian Laws of Eshnunna, 270
  passive prophylaxis, 273
  pets, 270
  post-exposure, 272–73
  precautions of vaccine, 274–75
  pre-exposure prophylaxis, 274
  pregnancy and, 64–65
  prevention, 272–74
  prodromal stage, 270–71
  Thomas on patient with, 270
  transmission, 271, 275
  treatment, 271
recombinant, adjuvanted zoster vaccine
  age limit, 168
  CDC recommending for people over 50, 168
  chemotherapy and, 170
  chickenpox or shingles prior to, 168–69
  discontinuation of live, attenuated zoster vaccine, 169
  effectiveness of Shingrix, 167
  immunization after case of shingles, 169
  patient (65 years) with underlying condition, 170
  Shingrix, 167
  varicella vaccine versus, 169–70
Recombivax HB, hepatitis B vaccine, 134
refugees, vaccine schedule, 97–98
reinfection, pertussis, 93
respiratory diphtheria, 74
  See also diphtheria
respiratory syncytial virus (RSV), 235–42
  active vaccinations, 239–40
  antigenic subtypes A and B, 236
  bovine RSV, 236
  chimpanzee coryza agent (CCA), 235
  clinical course, 237
  discovery, 235
  frequently asked questions, 240–42

INDEX

incubation period, 237
infant and mother vaccination, 71
infection, 235–36, 240
lethality of, 241
passive immunization, 238–39
pregnancy and, 60t, 64
prevention, 238–40
protecting newborn baby, 240–41
reinfections, 235–36, 241
risk factors for severe, 241–42
transmission, 236
treatment, 237
respiratory syncytial virus (RSV) vaccine(s)
contraindications, 240
dose and route of administration, 21t
nirsevimab (Beyfortus), 238
nirsevimab as "vaccine", 242
notes on adult immunization schedule, 39f
notes on child/adolescent immunization schedule, 29f
palivizumab (Synagis), 238–39
precautions of, 240
pregnancy and nirsevimab, 242
protection by nirsevimab, 242
RSVpreF (Pfizer), 239–40
RSVPreF3 (GlaxoSmithKline), 239
rifampin chemoprophylaxis, *Hemophilus influenzae* type b (Hib), 203–4
risk of vaccines, misconception on, 16–18
Roebling, John Augustus, tetanus death, 78
Roosevelt, Franklin D., polio, 208
rotaviruses, 216–22
adult infection, 221
age group and dosing, 47t
diarrheal illness, 216, 220
dose and route of administration, 21t
epidemiology of disease, 217
frequently asked questions, 220–22
incubation period, 218
infant vaccination, 20t, 221–22
pre-exposure, 218–19

prevention, 218–19
repeat infections, 220
segmented, double-stranded RNA viruses, 216–17
transmission, 217–18
vaccine contraindications, 219–20
vaccine efficacy, 220
vaccines and recommended use, 219t
worldwide infections, 216
rotavirus vaccines
age group and dosing (RSV), 47t
contraindications and precautions (live, attenuated oral), 223t
dose and route of administration (RSV), 21t
notes on child/adolescent immunization schedule, 29f
RSVpreF (Pfizer), 239–40
RSVPreF3 (GlaxoSmithKline), 239
RSV PreF3 vaccine, 21t
RSV preF vaccine, 21t
RV1--Rotarix, 223t
RV5--RotaTeq, 223t
rubella
clinical disease, 145–46
common anomalies, 146
complications, 146
congenital defects, 146
contraindications of MMR vaccine, 149
description of, 145
duration of protection, 148
frequently asked questions, 149–51
German measles, 145–46
immunogenicity, 148
incubation period, 147
MMR vaccine, 148
post-exposure, 147–48
precautions of MMR vaccine, 149
pre-exposure, 148
pregnancy and, 58, 65, 146
prevention, 147–48
transmission, 147
See also MMR (measles, mumps, rubella) vaccine

INDEX

rubeola (measles), pregnancy and, 64

safety, vaccine, 4-6
Salmonella species, typhoid fever, 261-62
SARS-CoV-2 (severe acute respiratory syndrome coronavirus 2), COVID-19, 58, 229, 230
screening blood test, hepatitis B virus (HBV), 131
sepsis, meningococcal, 183
serology screening, varicella, 163
sexual activity, HPV vaccination and, 199
sexual orientation, HPV vaccine and, 201
Shah of Iran (Shah Mohammed Reza Pahlavi), 85
shingles
   recombinant, adjuvanted zoster vaccine for adults over 50, 168-69
   varicella vaccination, 160
   See also herpes zoster
Shingrix
   effectiveness, 167
   frequently asked questions, 168-70
   recombinant, adjuvanted zoster vaccine, 167
   See also herpes zoster
smallpox, eradication of, ix, 3-4
smallpox vaccination
   ACAM2000 and JYNNEOS, 250, 252-53
   mpox immunization, 249
smokers
   pneumococcal vaccines, 178
   risk for pneumococcal disease, 173
snake venom, Buddhists, ix
South America, yellow fever, 255-57
Spanish influenza pandemic (1918), 99
splenectomy, elective
   Hib vaccines, 207
   pneumococcal vaccines and, 182
Staphylococcus aureus, 61-62, 101-2, 135-36

Sternberg, George, *Streptococcus pneumoniae*, 171
Streptococcus pneumoniae, 61-62, 101-2, 135-36
   identification of, 171
   risk factors, 67
subacute sclerosing panencephalitis (SSPE), 135-36
subcutaneous (SC) injection
   HPV vaccine and, 201
   injection site and needle size, 24t
swine flu vaccine, Guillain-Barré syndrome (GBS) and, 110

tack-borne encephalitis vaccine (TicoVax), 20t
Td (tetanus and diphtheria), 20t
   contraindications and precautions, 223t
Tdap (tetanus, diphtheria, acellular pertussis) vaccine, 2, 20t
   age group and dosing, 47t
   booster for cocoon effect, 97
   breastfeeding, 97
   contraindications and precautions, 223t
   encephalopathy, 92
   health care workers (HCWs), 93
   notes on adult immunization schedule, 39f
   notes on child/adolescent immunization schedule, 29f
   pertussis-containing vaccines, 90, 91
   pregnancy and, 59-61, 60t
   pregnant women, 96-97
   upper age limit for administration, 96
   visiting newborn grandchild and, 71
   See also tetanus, diphtheria, acellular pertussis (Tdap)
tetanus, ix, 2
   clinical forms, 79-80
   Clostridium tetani, 79, 80
   contraindications, 83
   duration of immunity, 83
   frequently asked questions, 83-85
   generalized, 79, 80

INDEX

incubation period, 80
"lockjaw", 79
neonatal, 79, 80
post-exposure, 81–82
precautions, 83
pre-exposure, 82
prevention, 81–82
routine health maintenance, 84
transmission, 80
wound management, 81, 81t
tetanus, diphtheria, acellular pertussis (Tdap). *See* Tdap (tetanus, diphtheria, acellular pertussis)
tetanus booster, vaccination record, 96
tetanus immune globulin (TIG), 81, 81t
wound management, 84
tetanus toxoid
vaccination of refugees or immigrants, 97–98
vaccines containing thimerosal, 14t
thimerosal
autism spectrum disorder (ASD) and, 150–51
mercury and, 12–13
safety in vaccines, 12–13
vaccines containing, 14t
Thomas, Lewis, on patient with rabies, 270
Thoreau, Henry David, brother John, 78
Thoreau, John, tetanus death, 78
tick-borne encephalitis (TBE)
Central European countries, 282–83
contraindications of vaccine, 285
duration of protection, 285
Estonia as endemic, 286–87
frequently asked questions, 286–87
human viral infection of central nervous system, 282–83
incubation period, 284
Ixodes ovatus, 282–83, 284
Ixodes persulcatus, 282–83, 284
Ixodes ricinus, 282–83, 284
neurotropic TBEV, 283
precautions of vaccine, 286
prevention, 284–85

primary vaccination schedule, 284–85
transmission, 284
travelers to Europe and Asia, 286
travel to Estonia, 286–87
tick-borne encephalitis vaccine (TicoVax), dose and route of administration, 21t
Tolstoy, Leo, pneumococcal pneumonia, 171
traveling abroad
hepatitis A vaccine and, 123–24
influenza vaccine and, 116
meningococcal vaccines, 192
See also yellow fever vaccine
Ty21a (Vivotif Berna, Swiss Serum and Vaccine Institute), typhoid fever vaccine, 263t
typhoid fever, 260–65
contraindications of vaccine, 264
diarrhea for infected persons, 102
frequently asked questions, 264–65
global health problem, 261–62
incubation period, 262
Mozart, 261
precautions of vaccine, 264
pre-exposure prophylaxis, 262
pregnancy and, 68
prevention, 262
Salmonella species, 261–62
transmission, 262
treatment, 262
"Typhoid Mary" (Mary Mallon), 260–61
vaccines, 263t

U.S. Food and Drug Administration (FDA)
safety of vaccines, 13
vaccine approval, 12

vaccination
concept of, ix
histories, xi
pertussis disease, 93

INDEX

vaccination record, tetanus booster and, 96
vaccination status, health care provider communication, 17–18
vaccine(s)
  addressing patient concerns, 3–19
  barriers to usage, xi–xii
  common, by type, 20t
  contraindications and precautions of commonly used, 223, 223t
  development of, x
  dose and route for administration, 21t
  facts on, 1–3
  frequently asked questions for pregnancy and, 70–71
  immunization schedule, 2
  immunological response to, 2
  inactivated, 1
  injection site and needle size, 24t
  live, attenuated, 1, 3
  misconception about toxins in, 12–15
  misconception on, as causing disease or infection, 18–19
  misconception on risk of, 16–18
  pregnancy and, 58–71, 60t
  recommendations by health care provider, 6–233
  reliable sources for information on, 18–19
  See also patient concerns about vaccines
vaccine-acquired immunity, misconception about natural immunity and, 11–12
Vaccine Adverse Event Reporting System (VAERS), 234–35
vaccine dose administration, age of person, 2
vaccine-preventable diseases (VPDs), x
  health care provider communication tip, 16
  health care provider communication tips, 11–12

  misconception of hygiene, sanitation, nutrition, and antibiotics and, 15–16
vaccine-preventable infections, misconception on vaccines and, 15–16
vaccine recommendation, Centers for Disease Control and Prevention (CDC), 3
vaccine safety, 4–6
  health care provider communication tips, 13–15
  misconception about toxins, 12–15
van Buren, Martin, 99
varicella, 20t
  dose and route of administration, 21t
  serology screening for, 163
varicella vaccine
  age group and dosing, 47t
  chickenpox exposure and, 159
  contraindications and precautions, 223t
  health professions and, 162
  immuno-compromised patients, 161
  infants traveling internationally, 159
  mild case of chickenpox and, 160
  minimum age for, 159
  natural and vaccine-acquired immunity, 11
  notes on adult immunization schedule, 39f
  notes on child/adolescent immunization schedule, 29f
  post-exposure setting, 163
  post-vaccination serologic testing, 163
  pregnancy and, 60t, 65–66
  recommendations for use in immunodeficient children, 161
varicella zoster, 7–8, 152–64
  appearance of rash, 153
  chickenpox, 152–64

INDEX

chickenpox vaccine in United States, 152
clinical course, 153–54
complications, 153–54
congenital varicella syndrome (fetal varicella syndrome), 154
contraindications of vaccine, 157–58
duration of protection, 157
effectiveness of vaccines, 157
frequently asked questions, 159–64
group A streptococcus, 153–54
hospitalizations and death before vaccination, 152
incubation period, 154–55
post-exposure, 155–56
precautions of vaccine, 158
pre-exposure, 156–57
pregnancy and, 156
prevention, 155–57
prophylactic administration of oral acyclovir or valacyclovir, 156
Staphylococcus aureus, 153–54
timing of maternal infection and potential outcome in fetus, 155*t*
transmission, 154
vaccine of susceptible persons, 156
varicella vaccines, 156–57
varicella zoster immune globulin (VariZIG) administration, 155
varicella zoster virus (VZV), 152–53
See also herpes zoster
varicella zoster immune globulin (VariZIG), infants, 163–64
varicella zoster vaccine, 7–8
Vibrio cholerae
oral ingestion of, 280
serogroups O1, 279
serogroups O1 and O139, 276–78
serogroups O1 El Tor, 276–78
ViCPS (Typhim Vi, Pasteur Merieux), typhoid fever vaccine, 263*t*

von Bismarck, Otto, herpes zoster (shingles), 164

Wakefield, Andrew, 7
Weissmuller, Johnny, polio, 208
West Africa, yellow fever, 255–57
whooping cough, pertussis, 85–86
Williams, Robin, herpes zoster (shingles), 164
World Health Organization (WHO), 276–78
  Region of Americas as polio-free, 209–10
World War I, 99
worldwide infants, unprotected, ix–x
wound management
  tetanus immune globulin (TIG), 84
  tetanus toxoid immunization history, 81, 81*t*
Wright, Sir Almroth, developing a vaccine for pneumococcal vaccine, 171

yellow fever (YF), 20*t*
  Aedes aegypti, 255, 257
  earliest record of, 255
  endemic areas of world, 255–57, 256*f*, 260
  incubation period, 257
  pregnancy and, 64, 71
  prevention, 258
  symptoms of, 255–57
  transmission, 257
  traveler's risk, 255–57
  treatment, 258
yellow fever vaccine, 255–60
  contraindications, 258
  duration of immunity, 258
  frequently asked questions, 259–60
  precautions, 259
  pre-exposure prophylaxis, 258
Young, Neil, polio, 208

INDEX

Zilber, L. A., tick-borne encephalitis (TBE), 283
zoster
    term, 164
    See also herpes zoster

zoster vaccine
    dose and route of administration, 21*t*
    health care employee, 162
    notes on adult immunization schedule, 39*f*